Sick, Spent, & 60 Nutrients Short

Why Your Doctor Treats the Symptoms While the Real Cause Goes Unchecked

Ravi Chimakurthy

Engineer | Systems Analyst | Product Manager | Nutrition Researcher

First Edition

Published by Cofactor Press

First Edition · 2026

ISBN: 979-8-9970108-1-2

Medical Disclaimer

This book is intended for educational and informational purposes only and does not constitute medical advice, diagnosis, or treatment. The nutritional information, reference ranges, dosage citations, and clinical discussions contained herein are drawn from published scientific research and are presented to inform and educate — not to replace the individualized assessment, diagnosis, or guidance of a qualified healthcare professional.

Nothing in this book should be interpreted as a recommendation to self-diagnose, self-treat, or discontinue any prescribed medication or treatment. Always consult your physician or a qualified healthcare professional before making any changes to your diet, supplementation, or treatment plan — particularly if you are pregnant, nursing, taking prescription medications, or managing a chronic health condition.

The statements in this book have not been evaluated by the Food and Drug Administration (FDA), the Therapeutic Goods Administration (TGA), the Medicines and Healthcare products Regulatory Agency (MHRA), or equivalent regulatory bodies in other jurisdictions. This book is not intended to diagnose, treat, cure, or prevent any disease.

For every patient who left a consultation room

with answers that did not match their questions.

And for the physicians who kept asking upstream

when the system rewarded downstream.

—

For my father, Gandhi Raja Chimakurthy,

who always believed in me,

who gave me the love of reading

and a keen sense of observation — the two things that made this book possible.

And for my father-in-law, Krishna Mohan Kantety,

physician, who had the patience his patients deserved —

who listened, who looked upstream,

and who understood, long before this book existed,

that what a patient eats matters as much as what a patient takes.

—

For my daughters, Neha and Nesta,

who inspired these pages by leaving the room every time I mentioned nutrition —

this book was always for you first.

And for my wife, Haritha,

who told me to write it for the world,

who told me to finish it when I hesitated,

and who told me, with characteristic honesty,

that the first version was too technical for the people who needed it most.

She was right on all three counts.

And for my mother, Lalitha Kumari, and for my dear friend, Martha Shultheis,

who were always all ears —

my first audience, across all the years,

whenever I had something to say about nutrition.

A Note on Method

This book was researched and written with the assistance of Claude, an artificial intelligence developed by Anthropic, used as a tool for synthesizing published scientific literature and for drafting across multiple disciplines. As with any source, readers are encouraged to verify information against the primary references cited and to consult qualified healthcare professionals.

Table of Contents

The Fourteen Clusters

The Synthesis

Preface

Why I Wrote This Book

This book was written for everyone who has sat in a doctor's office, received a diagnosis, been handed a prescription, and left still not knowing why. It was written from two decades of asking that question across three continents — in waiting rooms and consultation suites in India, Australia, and America — and watching the same scene repeat with remarkable consistency.

A doctor enters. A diagnosis is delivered — fluent, confident, wrapped in Latin. A prescription follows. And the appointment ends, usually within fifteen minutes, with the question that matters most still unasked: not what is wrong, but why.

I asked that question often. The responses taught me as much as any medical journal. Some physicians went in circles, retreating into genetics or environmental factors as conversation-enders rather than starting points for investigation. Some cited institutional protocols as though protocol were the same thing as explanation. A few, to their credit, admitted they simply did not know. To be fair, medicine answers the why with genuine confidence when the cause is infectious, traumatic, or toxic — the agent is identified, the mechanism is clear, the treatment follows logically. It is when the cause is nutritional and systemic that the question goes unanswered, the mechanism goes unexplored, and the consultation moves swiftly to the prescription pad. What none of them did — not once, across three countries and two decades — was ask about my diet. Not one inquired about what I ate, what I might be deficient in, or whether the nutrients required to run the biological systems in question were actually present in adequate supply. The prescription pad came out. The upstream cause stayed invisible.

I heard the same story from family, friends, and colleagues across every country I lived in. The pattern was identical everywhere: clinicians skilled at naming what was wrong and trained to treat its symptoms, but with no framework for asking why the system had failed in the first place. This is not a criticism of individual physicians. They operate inside a structure — specializations that function in silos, billing codes that reward throughput, consultation windows too narrow for root-cause inquiry. The system was not designed to look upstream. It was designed to manage downstream.

• • •

What Modern Medicine Stopped Asking

That question made me curious. Curiosity became research. Research became, over two decades, something closer to a vocation.

I began reading the current literature on nutritional biochemistry, then worked backward into the history of nutritional medicine — the ancient diseases that devastated populations, the pioneers who traced them to single nutrient deficiencies, and the resistance those pioneers faced from medical establishments unwilling to accept that chemistry, not contagion, was the cause. Joseph Goldberger proving that pellagra was a dietary deficiency disease, not an infectious one — a conclusion so threatening to the medical consensus of his day that even his self-experiments could not persuade it. James Lind demonstrating through one of history's first controlled clinical trials that citrus prevented scurvy, nearly two centuries before Albert Szent-Györgyi isolated the molecule responsible — ascorbic acid — and explained why. Roger Williams demonstrating that biochemical individuality meant optimal nutrition was not one-size-fits-all, but as individual as a fingerprint.

These discoveries were made. They were validated. And then, in the march of pharmaceutical medicine, they were quietly set aside — filed under 'solved' when the solution was only partial. Cereal fortification addressed the acute deficiency syndromes. It did not address the subclinical insufficiencies that persist in modern populations — insufficiencies that present not as pellagra or scurvy, but as fatigue, cognitive fog, metabolic dysfunction, disordered immunity, and the long cascade of chronic conditions that now constitute the primary burden of disease in the industrial world.

The assumption that deficiency diseases belong to the past is one of the most consequential errors in modern medicine. They did not disappear. They changed their clothes.

• • •

The Pattern That Kept Emerging

As the research accumulated, a pattern emerged that I could not ignore. Sixty nutrients. Fourteen biological systems. A web of dependencies so intricate, so interconnected, that no single specialist — looking only at the organ or system within their domain — could ever see it whole. A cardiologist sees the heart. An endocrinologist sees the thyroid. A neurologist sees the brain. None of them is looking at the common upstream substrate that all three depend on: the nutritional environment inside the cell.

The result is a patient — let us call her Margaret — who arrives at the medical system carrying fatigue, weight she cannot shift, a mood that will not lift, joints that ache without clear cause, immunity that fails too often, hormones that are out of range, and a cognitive edge that has quietly dulled. She sees five specialists. She leaves with five diagnoses and, eventually, five prescriptions. Nobody asks what Margaret eats. Nobody measures what Margaret's cells actually have to work with. Nobody considers that the five presentations might be one problem, expressed across five systems simultaneously.

The sixty nutrients in this book are not a list of supplements. They are the molecular inputs that Margaret's biology was designed to receive — inputs that industrial food has systematically stripped away in the name of shelf life, economics, and aesthetic consistency. What remains on Margaret's plate is calorie-dense and nutrient-empty. Her cells are running on fuel without the biochemical tools to use it properly.

• • •

The Invisible Famine Hypothesis

The insight that unified everything came not from a laboratory, but from observation across three continents.

I had spent years looking at two populations that appear, on the surface, to be opposites: the chronically malnourished in the developing world, and the chronically overfed in the industrial world. One population had too little. The other had, in caloric terms, more than enough. Yet when I looked at the downstream consequences — the fatigue, the immune failure, the metabolic disorder, the systemic breakdown of organ function — I kept feeling the same thing looking at both. The suffering was different in degree and presentation, but it was coming from the same place. The same biological machinery was failing in the same direction.

The explanation, I came to believe, lies in evolutionary biochemistry.

For two million years, the human body evolved a precise early-warning system — not for calories, but for nutrients. Vitamins, minerals, amino acid cofactors, essential fatty acids: the molecular raw materials that every cell requires to function. When those materials fall short, the body reads the signal clearly: scarcity is here. Famine may be coming. Activate the ancient response.

That response is elegant and ruthless. Store what you can — convert surplus energy into fat and hold it against the lean months ahead. Then triage everything else. Power down the systems that are metabolically expensive but not immediately critical for survival. Reproduction can wait. Deep immune surveillance can wait. Optimal thyroid output, mitochondrial efficiency, neurotransmitter synthesis, connective tissue repair — all of it can wait. The body is not failing. It is being precisely, evolutionarily rational.

The problem is that this ancient system cannot distinguish between a true famine and a modern diet. When Margaret consumes processed food stripped of its micronutrient content — high in calories, low in everything else — her hypothalamus receives the same signal it would receive if the harvest had failed. The nutrient sensors do not register abundance. They register absence. The hunger signals persist despite a full stomach. And the famine machinery activates: eat more, store more, power down. Leptin is the hormone the body uses to tell the brain that energy stores are sufficient — the molecular signal for fullness. In a well-nourished body, this signal flows cleanly: rising fat stores trigger rising leptin, the hypothalamus responds, appetite quiets. But chronic micronutrient depletion disrupts this loop. The hypothalamus, already reading nutrient absence as scarcity, becomes progressively desensitized to leptin's message. The signal is sent louder and louder. The receiver stops responding. Margaret is neurochemically starving while her body continues storing fat — and no amount of willpower overrides a broken satiety circuit. The hunger is not weakness. It is biology doing exactly what two million years of evolution designed it to do.

Eating more does not help, because more of the same nutrient-empty food deepens the scarcity signal rather than resolving it.

The fat accumulation is the most visible result. But it is only the surface. Below it, systems are going dark one by one. Margaret is exhausted because her mitochondria are undersupplied with the B vitamins, CoQ10, magnesium, and trace minerals they require to generate ATP efficiently. She is low in mood because serotonin and dopamine synthesis depend on cofactors her diet no longer reliably provides. Her immunity is erratic because immune surveillance is a metabolically costly operation that the triage protocol has quietly deprioritized. Her hormones are disordered because reproduction ranks low in a body managing what it believes to be a nutritional emergency. Her sleep is poor, her cognition has lost its edge, her joints ache, her skin has changed. Each symptom arrives separately in the clinic. Each receives its own name, its own code, its own prescription. None receives its real explanation.

They are all speaking the same language. The body is not producing a catalogue of unrelated conditions. It is executing a single, coherent, evolutionarily ancient response to a nutritional environment it was never designed to encounter: abundance without nourishment.

I call this the *Invisible Famine Hypothesis*.

It is invisible because no one is starving. The shelves are full, the plates are loaded, the calories are abundant. The famine is not in the food supply. It is in the nutrient density — and that absence is invisible to the patient who feels only its consequences, to the physician who sees only its symptoms, and to a medical system that was never trained to look for it.

The Invisible Famine Hypothesis may be the most consequential blind spot in modern medicine. Not because the science is absent — it is not; the evidence runs decades deep across hundreds of peer-reviewed papers — but because the system was never configured to connect it. No single specialist sees the whole. No standard panel measures what matters most. And no consultation that lasts fifteen minutes will ever ask the question that could change everything: what is Margaret actually missing?

• • •

What This Book Is

This book is the answer to that question.

It is organized around sixty nutrients, grouped into fourteen functional clusters — not by chemistry, but by the biological systems they sustain and the failures their absence produces. Each cluster is, in the language of the Invisible Famine Hypothesis, a set of switches the famine response turned off. The science behind each one is well-established, often decades deep, and largely absent from the standard of care that Margaret encounters when she walks into a clinic carrying a list of symptoms that no single diagnosis will ever fully explain.

This is not a book of prescriptions. It does not tell you what to take or in what dose — those decisions belong between you and a clinician who is willing to look upstream. What it does is lay out the evidence: what each nutrient does, what its absence produces, what the research shows, and why the medical system has so consistently failed to act on what the science has long established.

The giants of nutritional medicine — Goldberger, Williams, Warburg, Cheraskin, Lonsdale, Price, Pauling, Hoffer — were right. Pauling, who coined the term orthomolecular medicine and argued that humans require far more of certain nutrients than conventional medicine acknowledges. Hoffer, who spent decades demonstrating that psychiatric conditions long dismissed as purely psychological had nutritional substrates that responded to targeted intervention. They were all right decades before the molecular mechanisms were fully understood, and the mechanisms, as they have been elucidated, have vindicated them. This book stands on their work, extends it into the present, and attempts to make it accessible to the patient it was always intended to serve.

Margaret is not broken. She is depleted.

And depletion, unlike disease, has a direction out.

Opening: The Map We Were Given

Why Modern Medicine Sees Diseases Without Seeing Patients, Treats Symptoms Without Finding Causes, and Mistakes Sophisticated Diagnostics for Genuine Understanding

> *"The doctor of the future will give no medicine, but will interest his patients in the care of the human frame, in diet, and in the cause and prevention of disease."*

— *Thomas Edison, 1903*

I. The Patient in the Room

You have already met Margaret. She is fifty-three years old, moderately overweight, and has been through the medical system thoroughly enough to have accumulated a small portfolio of diagnoses. She has been told she has hypertension, for which she takes a beta-blocker and an ACE inhibitor. She has been told she has hypothyroidism, for which she takes levothyroxine. She has a diagnosis of generalized anxiety disorder, managed with a low-dose SSRI. She sees a dermatologist annually for a chronic skin condition that waxes and wanes without ever fully resolving. She has complained to her primary care physician about fatigue for three years running; the blood work comes back within normal limits, and the conversation ends there. Her gums bleed when she brushes her teeth, a fact she mentions to her dentist, who recommends better flossing technique. She has been told her cholesterol is borderline, that her triglycerides are somewhat elevated, and that she should eat better and exercise more.

Margaret sees five physicians. She takes five medications. She spends, between co-pays, prescriptions, specialist visits, and laboratory tests, somewhere between three and five thousand dollars per year navigating a system that has given her five diagnoses and zero explanations. She is not cured. She is managed. She has been told, implicitly and explicitly, that her conditions are chronic, that they are expected to require medication indefinitely, and that the goal of treatment is control rather than resolution.

Nobody has asked Margaret what she eats. Nobody has measured her magnesium. Nobody has assessed her vitamin D status in the context of her fatigue and her anxiety. Nobody has connected her bleeding gums to her cardiovascular risk or considered whether both might reflect the same upstream insufficiency. Nobody has asked about her history of antibiotic use — the four courses she took for recurrent respiratory infections in her forties, each of which left her gut flora diminished and her immune education subtly altered — or the proton pump inhibitor she was prescribed three years ago for reflux and has been taking ever since, silently impairing her absorption of magnesium, B12, and zinc. Nobody has asked about the stress she has carried for the better part of a decade, or considered that chronic cortisol elevation has been steadily increasing her thiamine demand beyond what her processed-food diet has ever supplied. Nobody has taken a nutritional history in any systematic way — because no one in her care team was trained to do so, because the system was not designed to ask that question, and because the question, if asked, would not generate a prescription, a procedure, or a billable code.

Margaret is not a rare or unusual patient. She is the model patient in internal medicine and primary care across the developed world. The details change but the structure is the same: multiple diagnoses, multiple medications, persistent symptoms, no upstream investigation, no resolution. She is the patient this book is written for, and she is the patient that the medicine described in this book would approach entirely differently.

> *Modern medicine is extraordinarily good at identifying what is wrong and giving it a name. It is considerably less good at asking why it went wrong in the first place. The diagnosis is the destination. The journey that led to it — the months or years of nutritional depletion, metabolic drift, and systemic deterioration that preceded the first symptom — is almost never the subject of clinical inquiry.*

II. Two Ways of Seeing: Germ and Terrain

To understand how medicine arrived at Margaret's situation — how a profession devoted to healing came to manage disease rather than resolve it, to treat downstream symptoms rather than upstream causes, to prescribe molecules rather than restore systems — you have to go back to the nineteenth century and a debate that medicine believes it settled but in fact simply abandoned.

In the 1860s and 1870s, two competing frameworks for understanding disease were developing in parallel in Europe. One was germ theory, associated primarily with Louis Pasteur and Robert Koch: the proposition that specific infectious diseases are caused by specific microorganisms, that the organism invades a susceptible host, and that the disease is properly understood as the consequence of that invasion. The framework was enormously productive. It explained cholera, tuberculosis, anthrax, and rabies. It led directly to vaccines, to antiseptic surgery, to antibiotics. It is one of the great intellectual achievements in the history of science, and the lives it has saved are beyond counting.

The other framework is associated most prominently with Antoine Béchamp, a French chemist and contemporary of Pasteur, and was concerned with what Béchamp called the terrain — the internal environment of the body. Béchamp's argument, simplified, was that the host's condition was at least as important as the pathogen's presence in determining whether disease developed. A microorganism encountered by a robust, well-nourished, metabolically resilient host might produce no illness or mild illness. The same microorganism in a depleted, nutritionally compromised, metabolically stressed host might produce severe disease. The pathogen mattered. But so did the soil it landed in.

These frameworks are not mutually exclusive. A mature medicine would have held both simultaneously: acknowledging that pathogens cause specific diseases while also attending to the metabolic and nutritional conditions that determine host susceptibility and the body's capacity for recovery. The history of medicine, had it developed differently, might have pursued both lines of inquiry with equal rigor and equal institutional investment. It did not develop differently. Germ theory won not merely as a scientific proposition but as a cultural and institutional one. It won because it was more compatible with the emerging pharmaceutical industry: if disease is caused by a specific external agent, the appropriate medical response is a specific counter-agent, a drug. It won because it was more tractable to the reductionist experimental methods that were becoming the gold standard of biomedical research. It won because it produced dramatic, unambiguous victories that terrain theory, operating on timescales of years and through the diffuse medium of nutrition and lifestyle, could not easily match.

What the Terrain Argument Actually Claimed

It is important to be precise here, because the terrain vs germ theory debate has been appropriated by fringe movements that have distorted both positions beyond recognition. Anti-vaccine proponents have cited terrain theory as a reason to reject germ theory entirely. This is a misreading of both frameworks. The terrain argument does not claim that pathogens are irrelevant. It claims that host condition is also relevant — that the question why did this person get sick when exposed to this pathogen is a legitimate and important medical question alongside what pathogen made this person sick.

The evidence for the terrain argument, properly understood, is not fringe. It is mainstream epidemiology. Mortality from tuberculosis had declined by more than 90% in England and Wales before the introduction of antibiotics, driven by improvements in nutrition, sanitation, and living conditions that altered the susceptibility of the host population. Infectious disease mortality across the developed world was already falling steeply before the interventions that germ theory produced arrived to accelerate the decline. The pathogens did not change. The terrain did.

The COVID-19 pandemic provided a contemporary illustration. The same virus produced radically different outcomes in different people — age, obesity, vitamin D status, and metabolic health among the strongest predictors of severity. These are terrain variables. The virus mattered. But so did the soil.

> *According to contemporaneous accounts, Louis Pasteur in his final years acknowledged the importance of the terrain, reportedly saying: Bernard was right; the pathogen is nothing, the terrain is everything. Whether the attribution is precise is disputed by historians. What is not disputed is that the scientific community in the century following Pasteur behaved as if he had said exactly the opposite — as if the pathogen were everything and the terrain were irrelevant. The institutional legacy of germ theory was a medicine that treated the invader and ignored the soil it invaded.*

III. Written in Pencil, Not Ink

When modern medicine cannot explain why you are sick, it often reaches for genetics. Your cholesterol is high because of a familial variant. Your fatigue is mitochondrial. Your autoimmune disease is HLA-linked. The implication is clear: your suffering has a molecular alibi, and that alibi is your DNA.

It is a seductive explanation. And for a narrow category of conditions — single-gene disorders like Huntington's disease or phenylketonuria — it is largely correct. But for the vast ocean of chronic disease that consumes modern healthcare, the genetics defense does not hold up under cross-examination.

Most disease-associated genetic variants do not cause disease. They raise the odds. They narrow the margin. The gene loads the gun; something else pulls the trigger. That something else, as this book will argue at length, is almost always biochemical — and biochemistry is exquisitely sensitive to nutritional status.

Consider what many of these variants actually are: instructions for enzymes that require specific micronutrient cofactors to function. The MTHFR polymorphism doesn't sentence you to cardiovascular disease or depression — it increases your requirement for folate and B12. The SOD2 Val16Ala variant doesn't doom your mitochondria — it raises your need for manganese and antioxidant support. FUT2 variants don't condemn you to B12 deficiency — they signal that your absorption mechanism is less efficient and your intake must compensate. In each case, the genetic finding is not a verdict. It is a map — pointing directly toward a nutritional gap that medicine has declined to fill.

Epigenetics makes this case even more forcefully. Gene expression is not fixed. It is regulated, moment to moment, by the availability of methyl donors, zinc, selenium, vitamin D, and dozens of other nutrients that conventional medicine rarely measures and almost never optimizes. Your genome is not the sentence. It is the instrument. Nutrition is what plays it.

Bruce Ames, whose triage theory you will encounter throughout this book, demonstrated that when micronutrients are scarce, the body rations them — prioritizing immediate survival over long-term genomic integrity. What looks like genetic destiny is often simply a body operating without the raw materials it needs.

So when your physician tells you that your condition is genetic, hear what that may actually mean: your biochemistry has a narrower margin for nutritional insufficiency than average. That is not a dead end. That is the beginning of a more precise and actionable question — one this book is written to help you ask.

IV. The Flexner Report and the Reformation of Medicine

In 1910, a man named Abraham Flexner published a report commissioned by the Carnegie Foundation and supported by

John D. Rockefeller's General Education Board that would reshape American medicine more profoundly than any single event before or since. The Flexner Report evaluated 155 medical schools across the United States and Canada, and its findings were damning: most of the schools were inadequately funded, poorly staffed, scientifically underpowered, and graduating physicians whose training bore little relationship to the emerging science of medicine.

These criticisms were largely correct, and the reforms that followed were, in important respects, genuine improvements. Medical education was restructured around laboratory science, pathology, pharmacology, and the reductionist methods of experimental biomedicine. Schools that could not meet the new standards were closed. The number of medical schools in the United States fell from 155 to 31 within fifteen years. The profession was standardized, credentialed, and elevated.

What is less often discussed is what was excluded in the process. The new model of medical education, funded substantially by Rockefeller and Carnegie philanthropy, was built around a conception of disease as biochemical pathology amenable to pharmaceutical correction. Nutrition, physical medicine, herbal and botanical traditions, and what would later be called lifestyle medicine were systematically marginalized or excluded from the new curriculum. They were not excluded because they were proven ineffective. They were excluded because they were not compatible with the reductionist pharmaceutical model, and because the philanthropic interests funding the new medical schools had significant investments in the pharmaceutical industry that the model would create.

This is not a conspiracy theory. It is documented history, and it requires no assumption of malicious intent. John D. Rockefeller and Andrew Carnegie were men of their era who believed in industrial rationalization and standardization as the path to progress. They applied to medicine the same logic they had applied to oil and steel: eliminate inefficiency, standardize production, invest in scale. The result was a more scientifically rigorous medical profession. It was also a medical profession whose intellectual architecture was structured around a particular theory of disease and a particular set of therapeutic tools — and whose curriculum had been systematically pruned of the traditions that asked different questions.

What Was Left Out

The curriculum that emerged from the Flexner reforms devoted virtually no time to nutrition. This was not an oversight. It was a structural feature of a model that conceived of disease as the target of pharmaceutical intervention, and of the physician's role as diagnostician and prescriber rather than as guide to the conditions under which health is maintained. A physician trained in the Flexnerian model learned pharmacology, pathology, and the management of disease states. They did not learn, in any systematic way, the conditions required for those disease states not to develop.

The consequences compound over time. Each generation of physicians was trained by the previous generation, the curriculum reinforced by a research agenda funded by pharmaceutical companies with no interest in nutritional interventions. The system had a center of gravity, and that center was not nutrition.

The result, a century after Flexner, is a medical profession in which the average physician receives between nineteen and twenty-nine hours of nutrition education across four years of medical school — a figure that has been documented repeatedly in surveys of medical school curricula and that has barely changed in decades. A profession that sees patients for an average of seven to fifteen minutes per visit, with little time and no incentive to conduct a nutritional assessment. A profession that is extraordinarily skilled at identifying pathology and prescribing the agents that manage it, and genuinely underprepared to ask why the pathology developed in the first place.

> *It requires no malice and no conspiracy to explain why modern medicine does not ask nutritional questions. It requires only the recognition that a profession is shaped by its training, its incentives, its research funding, and its institutional culture — and that all four of these, for the better part of a century, have pointed in a direction that leads away from the upstream and toward the downstream.*

V. The Gold Standard and Its Blind Spots

The randomized controlled trial is the methodological crown jewel of modern evidence-based medicine, and for many of the questions medicine asks, it deserves that status. When you want to know whether a specific drug reduces the incidence of a specific outcome compared to placebo, the RCT is the right tool. It controls for confounding, it separates signal from noise, it provides a level of inferential clarity that no other study design matches. The medicine that emerged from the systematic application of RCT methodology is safer, more rigorous, and more accountable than what preceded it.

But the RCT is a tool, and every tool has the shape of the questions it can answer. The randomized controlled trial was designed for pharmaceutical evaluation: one intervention, one outcome, a defined time horizon, a homogeneous patient population. This design is structurally ill-suited to the evaluation of nutritional interventions, and understanding why is essential to understanding why the evidence base for nutrition appears weaker than it is, and why nutrition has been systematically disadvantaged in the competition for clinical credibility.

Why Nutrition Does Not Fit the RCT Model

A drug is a single molecule administered at a precise dose for a defined period, producing effects that can be measured against a placebo with reasonable confidence that the measured effect is attributable to the molecule in question. A nutrient is embedded in a diet, interacts with dozens of other nutrients, operates within a metabolic context that varies between individuals, produces effects that accumulate over years rather than weeks, and cannot be meaningfully double-blinded against a placebo in free-living subjects who can taste and feel what they are consuming. The

RCT's greatest strength — its isolation of a single variable — is precisely what makes it a poor fit for the study of nutrients that operate within systems.

Consider what it would mean to design an RCT for vitamin D equivalent to the trials that established statin efficacy. You would need to randomize thousands of subjects to a precise dose of vitamin D for a decade or more, measure cardiovascular outcomes, and attribute the difference to vitamin D. But your placebo group is not getting zero vitamin D — they are getting whatever their diet and sun exposure provide, which varies enormously between individuals. Your treatment group is getting supplemental D3 on top of variable baseline intake. You are not measuring the effect of vitamin D versus no vitamin D. You are measuring supplemental D3 on top of variable background levels, in a population whose genetic variation, magnesium status, and cofactor availability you have not controlled. The signal may be real and substantial, and the study may still fail to detect it.

This is not a hypothetical. It is the methodological reality behind the confusing results of vitamin D RCTs — results cited as evidence that vitamin D does not work. The failure to find a signal is not the same as the absence of one. Nutrition research has been paying for that confusion in credibility for decades.

The Reductionism Problem

Behind the RCT's limitations lies a deeper methodological assumption: reductionism. The conviction that complex systems can be understood by isolating and manipulating single variables. In physics and chemistry, reductionism is extraordinarily productive. In the study of living systems — where everything interacts with everything else, where the effect of any intervention depends on the context in which it is applied, where the whole is genuinely more than the sum of its parts — reductionism is productive up to a point and then systematically misleading.

A nutrient does not act in isolation. Vitamin D requires magnesium. Niacin requires riboflavin. Vitamin C regenerates vitamin E. Thiamine requires magnesium for activation. B12 requires folate to function in methylation. Every nutrient this book discusses is embedded in a network of dependencies, and the effect of any single nutrient intervention depends on the status of the network it enters. An RCT that tests vitamin C in isolation, without measuring or controlling baseline ascorbate status, oxidative stress burden, cofactor availability, and dietary background, is testing vitamin C in a methodological vacuum. The null result it may produce tells you almost nothing about whether vitamin C matters.

Medicine has not failed to study nutrition. It has studied nutrition with tools designed for a different kind of question and concluded, from the resulting noise, that nutrition is not amenable to rigorous study. The conclusion is backward. Nutrition is not the problem. The methodology is.

VI. The Specialist Trap: When Nobody Owns the Upstream

Modern medicine is organized around specialties, and the specialties are organized around organ systems and disease categories. The cardiologist manages the heart. The neurologist manages the nervous system. The gastroenterologist manages the gastrointestinal tract. The psychiatrist manages the mind. Each specialty has its own training pathways, its own journals, its own clinical guidelines, its own therapeutic toolkit. The organization is logical, efficient, and, for the management of specific organ-system pathology within well-defined categories, genuinely effective.

But it has a structural blind spot the size of a continent: it has no mechanism for asking whether pathology in multiple organ systems simultaneously might reflect a single upstream cause. The upstream question — why is this happening in multiple systems at once? — is nobody's job. It is not taught in any specialty curriculum. It is not reimbursed by any billing code. It is not the subject of any specialty guideline. It falls into the space between the silos, and in that space, patients like Margaret accumulate diagnoses.

The Polypharmacy Consequence

The specialist trap produces a predictable downstream consequence: polypharmacy. When five specialists each see one component of a multi-system syndrome and each prescribes the agent indicated for their component, the patient goes home with five medications. Each medication was rationally indicated for its target condition. The combination may interact. The drugs may deplete nutrients. Several drugs commonly prescribed for the conditions Margaret carries — beta-blockers, ACE inhibitors, proton pump inhibitors, SSRIs — have documented effects on nutrient status that are essentially never discussed in clinical encounters.

Beta-blockers deplete coenzyme Q10, the mitochondrial electron carrier that cardiac muscle depends on for its prodigious energy requirements — a depletion that may worsen the very cardiac function the drug is prescribed to support. Proton pump inhibitors, by suppressing gastric acid, impair the absorption of magnesium, vitamin B12, iron, and zinc — the very nutrients whose deficiency produces fatigue, neuropathy, and impaired immune function. SSRIs have documented effects on folate metabolism. ACE inhibitors affect zinc status. Loop diuretics deplete thiamine and potassium. The medications prescribed to manage Margaret's conditions are, as a pharmacological side effect, deepening the nutritional insufficiency that may have contributed to her conditions in the first place. Nobody is tracking this. Nobody has been asked to.

The following table documents the most clinically significant drug-nutrient depletion interactions — the nutritional costs of the pharmaceutical management that millions of patients like Margaret receive without anyone connecting the prescription to the deficiency:

Common Drug Class	Nutrient(s) Depleted	Potential Consequence of Depletion
Beta-blockers	Coenzyme Q10	Reduced cardiac and mitochondrial energy production; worsened fatigue; exercise intolerance; may worsen the heart failure the drug is prescribed to prevent
Proton pump inhibitors (PPIs)	Magnesium, vitamin B12, iron, zinc	Fatigue, peripheral neuropathy, impaired immunity, increased fracture risk, cognitive decline; FDA issued magnesium warning in 2011 — largely unimplemented in clinical monitoring
Loop diuretics (furosemide, bumetanide)	Thiamine, potassium, magnesium, calcium, zinc	Cardiac dysfunction, peripheral nerve impairment, muscle cramps, arrhythmia risk; the thiamine depletion may worsen the heart failure the diuretic is treating — a documented iatrogenic loop
Thiazide diuretics (HCTZ, chlorthalidone)	Magnesium, potassium, zinc, sodium	Muscle weakness, cardiac arrhythmia, insulin resistance, fatigue; potassium depletion is routinely monitored; magnesium depletion is not, despite being equally clinically significant
Statins	Coenzyme Q10	Myopathy (muscle pain and weakness in 5–20% of users); fatigue; reduced mitochondrial function; may worsen heart failure through CoQ10 depletion in the cardiac muscle the statin is intended to protect
Metformin	Vitamin B12,	Peripheral neuropathy; elevated

Common Drug Class	Nutrient(s) Depleted	Potential Consequence of Depletion
	folate	homocysteine; cognitive decline; megaloblastic anemia; B12 depletion is undermonitored — ADA recommends periodic B12 assessment in long-term metformin users
ACE inhibitors	Zinc	Impaired immune function, poor wound healing, taste disturbance; zinc depletion may contribute to the chronic cough that is the most common reason ACE inhibitors are discontinued
Oral contraceptives	B6, B12, folate, zinc, magnesium, vitamin C	Mood dysregulation, depression, impaired methylation cycle, immune suppression; the folate depletion is particularly significant if pregnancy follows discontinuation
SSRIs	Folate (indirectly, through interaction with folate-dependent methylation pathways)	Impaired methylation cycle; may blunt antidepressant treatment response — the reason some patients respond better when folate or methylfolate is added to their SSRI regimen
Corticosteroids	Vitamin C, calcium, vitamin D, zinc, magnesium, potassium	Impaired immunity, bone loss (osteoporosis with prolonged use), wound healing failure, adrenal suppression; calcium and vitamin D supplementation is sometimes co-prescribed but vitamin C, zinc, and magnesium depletion are not addressed
Anticonvulsant	Vitamin D,	Bone demineralization,

Common Drug Class	Nutrient(s) Depleted	Potential Consequence of Depletion
s (phenytoin, carbamazepine, valproate)	B12, folate, biotin, vitamin K	peripheral neuropathy, impaired clotting, neural tube risk in pregnancy; patients on long-term anticonvulsants require comprehensive fat-soluble and B-vitamin monitoring
H2 blockers (famotidine, cimetidine)	Vitamin B12, iron, zinc	Similar to PPIs though generally milder — achlorhydria from H2 blockade reduces mineral solubilization and intrinsic factor-dependent B12 absorption; B12 deficiency with prolonged use
Antibiotics (broad-spectrum)	Vitamin K2, B vitamins (via microbiome disruption)	Impaired coagulation factor carboxylation; reduced bacterial B-vitamin synthesis; gut dysbiosis with downstream consequences for immunity, mood, and nutrient absorption — effects may persist for months after a single course
NSAIDs (chronic use)	Vitamin C, iron (via gastrointestinal bleeding), folate	Gut permeability and mucosal damage; iron deficiency anemia from occult GI bleeding; impaired antioxidant defense through vitamin C depletion; folate loss from mucosal cell turnover

VII. The Curriculum Gap: What Physicians Are Not Taught

In 2010, a survey published in Academic Medicine found that only 27% of American medical schools met the minimum recommended 25 hours of nutrition education. A 2015 survey found that the average medical student received 19.6 hours of nutrition instruction across four years of training — roughly the same amount of time devoted to a single pharmacology module. A 2019 survey of graduating medical students found that fewer than 20% felt adequately prepared to counsel patients on nutrition.

These numbers have not meaningfully changed in thirty years of surveys, despite repeated calls for reform from nutrition scientists, dietitians, and a minority of physicians who recognize the gap. The curriculum does not change because the institutional forces that shape it — faculty priorities, accreditation standards, licensing examination content, and the research interests of academic medical departments — do not assign nutrition a priority that would drive curricular change. Pharmacology receives substantially more teaching time than nutrition in virtually every American medical school. This is not because drugs are more important to health than food. It is because the institutional structures that fund and shape medical education have, for a century, treated them that way.

The consequence is a profession that is genuinely well-equipped to recognize and manage established disease and genuinely underprepared to recognize the nutritional antecedents of disease or to intervene in the long pre-clinical period when nutritional restoration might prevent the disease from developing. The physician who sees Margaret does not ask about her diet not because they are uncurious or negligent but because they were never taught what to ask, were never shown how to interpret what they might find, and are operating within a system that provides no time, no reimbursement, and no clinical pathway for nutritional investigation.

This is not a criticism of individual physicians. It is a structural observation about the system that trains them, rewards them, and defines the boundaries of their practice. The physicians in this book's story — Goldberger, Lonsdale, Hoffer, Pauling, Cameron — were, in various ways, physicians who stepped outside those boundaries. They were not rewarded for it. The boundaries have not moved.

VIII. The Economics of Downstream: Why the System Treats Symptoms

It would be convenient, for the purposes of a satisfying narrative, to identify a villain in this story. A room of executives who decided to prioritize profit over health. A regulatory agency captured by industry. A professional association that knowingly suppressed inconvenient evidence. These elements exist, in varying degrees, and they are not irrelevant. But they are not the primary explanation for why medicine treats symptoms rather than causes, and attributing the system's failures primarily to malice obscures the more mundane and more intractable reality: the system treats symptoms because that is what it was designed to do, and the design reflects incentives that, individually rational at every node, produce collectively irrational outcomes at the level of population health.

Consider the economics of a chronic disease. A patient with hypertension who takes an antihypertensive medication for thirty years generates thirty years of prescription revenue, thirty years of monitoring visits, thirty years of laboratory tests, and, eventually, a higher-than-average probability of the cardiovascular event that generates the most intensive and expensive medical intervention of all. A patient with hypertension whose blood pressure normalizes over twelve months through magnesium repletion, vitamin D optimization, dietary change, and thiamine sufficiency — interventions that cost a fraction of thirty years of pharmaceutical management — generates a small, time-limited revenue stream and then exits the system as a resolved case. From the perspective of the patient, this is the ideal outcome. From the perspective of a healthcare economy built around the management of chronic disease, it represents a lost revenue stream.

This is not a conspiracy. It is an incentive structure. No individual physician wakes up planning to keep patients sick for revenue. No pharmaceutical executive explicitly designs trials to produce null results for nutritional interventions. What happens instead is subtler and more pervasive: the system funds the research that serves its interests, trains physicians in the interventions that generate revenue, reimburses the treatments that maintain chronic conditions, and systematically defunds, dismisses, and marginalizes the interventions that might resolve them. The outcome — a medicine that manages disease more effectively than it prevents or cures it — is not designed. It is emergent. It is the predictable result of a century of incentive alignment pointing in a consistent direction.

> *The United States spends approximately 4.5 trillion dollars per year on healthcare. In the World Health Organization's landmark 2000 assessment, it ranked thirty-seventh in the world in health outcomes. The gap between expenditure and outcome is not a mystery. It is the arithmetic of a system that has confused the treatment of disease with the pursuit of health, and that has invested with extraordinary generosity in the former while neglecting the latter almost entirely.*

The Research Funding Problem

The distortion in clinical practice is upstream funded by a distortion in research. The National Institutes of Health allocates the majority of its research budget to disease mechanisms and pharmaceutical interventions. The proportion allocated to nutritional research has remained a small fraction of the total, and much of what is allocated goes to large epidemiological studies whose observational design cannot establish causation — the very design limitation that critics then cite as evidence that nutrition research is inherently weak.

The pharmaceutical industry funds approximately sixty percent of clinical trial research in the United States, and industry-funded trials are more likely to reach positive conclusions for the sponsored product — a documented, replicated finding requiring no assumption of fraud. Nutritional interventions cannot be patented, cannot generate the returns that justify billion-dollar clinical trial programs, and therefore are not studied at the scale that pharmaceutical interventions are studied. They do not accumulate comparable evidence, and the profession then applies equal evidentiary standards to interventions studied at radically unequal scales of investment. The game is played on a tilted field, and the profession declares the losers inferior on the basis of the score.

IX. The Deficiency Pattern Nobody Is Looking For

There is a pattern running through the history of medicine that has been identified, celebrated in the specific, and ignored in the general. The pattern is this: a complex, multi-system disease that has baffled the profession for years is eventually traced to the deficiency of a single essential nutrient. The finding produces a Nobel Prize or its equivalent, a period of clinical excitement, a public health intervention, and then a filing away of the case as solved and closed. The general lesson — that complex, multi-system disease can have simple, upstream, nutritional causes — is never extracted from the specific case and applied as a diagnostic principle.

Scurvy was one such case. The bleeding gums, the reopening wounds, the fatal hemorrhages of sailors at sea were traced to vitamin C deficiency, and the diagnosis that had mystified the medical establishment for two centuries was resolved by citrus fruit. The lesson: collagen-dependent tissues fail when vitamin C is absent. Application to the modern world: negligible. Beriberi was another. The paralysis, the heart failure, the neurological devastation of populations eating polished rice were traced to thiamine deficiency. The lesson: when the cofactor for the primary gateway enzyme of aerobic metabolism is absent, every high-energy-demand tissue fails simultaneously. Application to the modern world: negligible. Pellagra was a third. The dermatitis, the diarrhea, the dementia of the American South were traced to niacin deficiency, and Goldberger's heroic epidemiology resolved in a decade what the germ theorists had failed to resolve in thirty years. Application to the modern world: negligible.

In each case, the solved disease continues to exist in subtler, subclinical forms — insufficiency rather than deficiency, functional impairment rather than frank pathology — in populations whose diet does not produce dramatic beriberi or pellagra but whose nutrient status falls far short of what the biological evidence suggests is optimal. These subclinical forms are not rare. They are among the most prevalent and most consequential health conditions of the modern era. They are simply not recognized as such because the diagnostic framework built to identify frank deficiency disease was never extended to subclinical insufficiency.

Sixty Nutrients, One Pattern

The vitamins are the most familiar members of the category of essential non-caloric nutrients — the micronutrients that the body requires in small amounts to perform specific biochemical functions and cannot synthesize in adequate amounts independently. But the category is larger and less well-known than the vitamin story alone. It includes the minerals: macro-minerals like magnesium, calcium, potassium, phosphorus, and sulfur, and trace minerals like zinc, iron, copper, selenium, manganese, molybdenum, chromium, iodine, boron, vanadium, and silica. It includes conditionally essential compounds like coenzyme Q10, carnitine, and alpha-lipoic acid. It includes the essential fatty acids. It includes the amino acids that are essential or conditionally essential — those the body cannot synthesize at all, and those it cannot synthesize in adequate amounts under conditions of metabolic stress.

Together, these nutrients number approximately sixty in the category that this book examines. They are not independent variables. They form a web of interdependencies in which each nutrient's function is conditioned by the availability of others, in which the deficiency of one creates increased demand for several others, and in which the cumulative effect of multiple simultaneous insufficiencies is not the sum of their individual effects but something qualitatively different. It is a broad metabolic impairment that touches every system and produces a clinical picture of chronic, multi-system dysfunction that looks nothing like the textbook deficiency diseases because it is not a textbook deficiency disease. It is something subtler, more diffuse, more modern, and in some ways more dangerous precisely because it is invisible to the diagnostic framework that was built to identify something else.

This is the pattern this book is about. Not a single nutrient deficiency producing a dramatic clinical syndrome. But a web of insufficiencies, each below the threshold of clinical recognition, collectively producing the chronic disease burden of the developed world. Not scurvy. Something that looks like cardiovascular disease, fatigue, anxiety, and inflammatory conditions. Not beriberi. Something that looks like dysautonomia, heart failure with preserved ejection fraction, and irritable bowel syndrome. Not pellagra. Something that looks like treatment-resistant depression, chronic skin conditions, and metabolic syndrome. The names are different. The upstream logic is the same.

This is why the book you are holding is not organized the way every nutritional book before it has been organized. A chapter on magnesium that does not explain why magnesium deficiency makes thiamine non-functional tells an incomplete story. A chapter on thiamine that does not show how copper deficiency at the far end of the same energy pathway produces identical consequences is a fragment masquerading as a whole. A chapter on selenium that does not connect it to the iodine it activates, the glutathione it regenerates, and the thyroid autoimmunity it modulates has described one musician in an orchestra and called it a performance. The sixty nutrients in this book are grouped into fourteen clusters — not because the grouping is arbitrary or convenient, but because the biology demands it. The dependency between these nutrients is not a footnote. It is the argument.

X. Our Ancestral Diet

The diet that assembled this nutrient framework was not designed. It carried no philosophy, no label, and no calorie targets. It was the sum of what was available — and what was available, across most of human evolutionary history, happened to cover virtually every biological need simultaneously. The ancestral diet was nutritionally complete by accident of circumstance, not by intention. It rested on four pillars that modern diets have quietly dismantled, one by one.

The first pillar was **the whole animal** — organ meats, muscle, bone marrow, fat, skin, and tendon. The second was **seasonal diverse plants** — hundreds of wild species rotating through the year, bitter, fibrous, and geographically diverse in ways the modern produce aisle is not. The third was **fruits in season** — not year-round, not hybridized for sweetness, genuinely nutrient-dense rather than the calorie-forward varieties bred for shelf life and palatability. The fourth was **nuts and seeds** — foraged across dozens of species, unprocessed, eaten in natural quantities. No one counted nutrients because none were missing. Completeness was the default, not the achievement.

I. The Whole Animal Principle

The parts that modern diets discard were the parts most prized. Liver, kidney, heart, bone marrow, brain. Each organ is a concentrated depot of the nutrients that organ requires to function — which is precisely why eating it transfers those nutrients efficiently to the organism that consumes it. This was not cultural preference. It was nutritional logic operating without the science to name it.

Liver delivers retinol, copper, B12, choline, iron, folate, and CoQ10 in concentrations that no plant food approaches and no modern supplement combination fully replicates. Heart muscle is the densest dietary source of coenzyme Q10. Kidney provides selenium, B12, and heme iron at densities that muscle meat cannot match. Bone marrow delivers fat-soluble vitamins and the glycine-rich collagen precursors that joint, skin, and connective tissue synthesis depend on. The abandonment of organ meats in modern Western diets was not a neutral dietary shift. It quietly removed the most nutrient-dense foods humans had consumed across most of their evolutionary history — with no systematic replacement plan and no clinical recognition of the gap it opened.

II. The Plant Diversity Collapse

Hunter-gatherers consumed an estimated 150 to 200 plant species annually. The modern diet runs on roughly twelve. The polyphenol, carotenoid, and phytonutrient coverage that the final cluster of this book documents was delivered automatically by seasonal rotation across hundreds of wild plant varieties — bitter, fibrous, colorful, and geographically diverse in ways that the modern supermarket vegetable section is not. Wild fruits were smaller, less sweet, and more phytonutrient-dense than the hybridized varieties bred for palatability and year-round availability. Wild nuts and seeds were foraged across dozens of species rather than drawn from a short list of commercially cultivated options. The modern produce aisle is a narrow, sweetened, and domesticated extract of that ancestral range — optimized for yield, shelf life, and consumer preference rather than for the breadth of biological signals the body evolved to receive.

III. The Conditionally Essential Reclassification

Several compounds in this book carry the designation "conditionally essential" — a classification that deserves closer examination than nutritional science has given it. Taurine, carnitine, coenzyme Q10, creatine, and glycine are categorized as non-essential because the body can synthesize them endogenously. The classification is technically accurate. It is also historically contingent in a way that has never been properly acknowledged.

The classification was established in populations that ate organ meats, muscle meat, and fish regularly — populations in which dietary intake of these compounds was constant, abundant, and assumed. Endogenous synthesis was not required to carry the full load, because dietary top-up was always arriving. Remove the dietary top-up — as modern diets largely have, and plant-based diets completely do — and endogenous synthesis becomes the entire supply chain. It was not designed to carry that load alone. The result is a slow, systemic undersupply that blood tests rarely capture, that physicians were never taught to suspect, and that the "non-essential" label makes invisible by definition.

The "non-essential" label is not a biological absolute. It is a historically contingent classification that quietly became obsolete the moment modern diets eliminated the foods that made it valid. For the patient who no longer eats organ meats, no longer eats fish, and lives on a food supply that has optimized for calories rather than nutrients, taurine, carnitine, CoQ10, creatine, and glycine are functionally essential — and functionally absent. The consequences appear in the clinic under other names — fatigue, depression, cardiac dysfunction, cognitive decline — and leave with prescriptions that address none of their upstream cause.

IV. The Modern Diet Failure Matrix

Every contemporary dietary pattern, however carefully constructed, leaves something out. The standard Western diet displaces nutrient density almost entirely with processed, calorie-dense food. The "healthy" Western diet — whole grains, lean proteins, abundant vegetables — closes many gaps but leaves copper, CoQ10, taurine, and K2 largely unaddressed, because the organ meats that supplied them have been removed without replacement. The lacto-ovo vegetarian diet closes B12 and retinol partially through eggs and dairy, but cannot reliably supply taurine, carnitine, CoQ10, creatine, or DHA. The vegan diet compounds every one of these gaps and adds B12, heme iron, zinc bioavailability, and iodine to the list. The carnivore diet, moving in the opposite direction, eliminates polyphenols, carotenoids, vitamin C, and the prebiotic fiber on which the microbiome depends. The Mediterranean diet — routinely cited as the gold standard of evidence-based dietary guidance — performs better than most, but organ meats are largely absent from its modern practice, and with them go copper, CoQ10, and taurine.

Even the Paleo diet — the dietary framework most consciously modeled on ancestral eating — falls short of the ancestral baseline, because the food supply itself has changed. Grain-fed meat is not wild ruminant. Farmed salmon is not wild salmon. Supermarket eggs are not the eggs of hens foraging freely on insects, grubs, and diverse plant matter. The animals that modern diets draw from are themselves nutritionally depleted relative to their wild counterparts, having been raised on diets as narrow and processed as the humans who will eventually eat them.

No modern diet achieves what ancestral eating delivered by default. Everyone is a partial reconstruction. Some gaps are small. Some are systemic. All are invisible to the medicine that treats their consequences as independent diseases.

V. The Three-Level Famine

The Invisible Famine described in this book does not operate at a single level. It compounds across three simultaneously, and the ancestral diet operated cleanly at all three without effort.

The first level is **food choice**: the exclusion from modern diets of the most nutrient-dense foods that the four ancestral pillars provided. The second is **food quality**: depleted soils, grain-fed animals, hybridized crops, and processing losses that strip nutrients from even the right foods before they reach the plate. The third is **absorption**: gut dysbiosis, pharmaceutical burden, chronic inflammation, and reduced stomach acid that impair the uptake of whatever nutrients do arrive. Modern diets struggle at all three levels simultaneously. The gap between dietary intention and nutritional outcome is wider than medicine has acknowledged — and wider than most patients suspect.

Every modern diet is an attempt to reconstruct from fragments what ancestral eating delivered whole. The reconstruction is necessary — we cannot and should not eat precisely as our ancestors did. But reconstruction without a map leaves gaps. Gaps that accumulate. Gaps that medicine treats as diseases. The fourteen clusters that follow are that map.

XI. How to Read This Book

This book is not an argument that medicine is wrong. It is an argument that medicine is incomplete. The physicians who trained in the Flexnerian model, who practice evidence-based medicine according to the guidelines of their specialty, who prescribe the agents that clinical trials have shown to be effective — they are doing what they were trained to do, and much of what they do is genuinely valuable. The cardiologist who manages acute myocardial infarction with thrombolytics and interventional cardiology is practicing a form of medicine that saves lives that would otherwise be lost, and this book does not dispute that.

What this book disputes is the completeness of that medicine as a model for health. The cardiologist who saves the heart attack patient with a stent has accomplished something real and important. The cardiologist who then prescribes a statin, a beta-blocker, and an ACE inhibitor and considers the case managed has accomplished something real but incomplete. The question of why the coronary artery developed the plaque that caused the event — the decade-long upstream story of oxidative stress, vitamin C insufficiency and failed collagen cross-linking (Cluster 5), the omega-6-driven inflammatory membrane environment (Cluster 13), magnesium depletion impairing both ATP synthesis and endothelial function (Cluster 1), and the methylation impairment allowing homocysteine to damage the arterial wall (Cluster 9) — has not been asked, and the interventions that might address it have not been offered.

Each cluster in this book brings together a group of nutrients that operate as an integrated section of the orchestra — nutrients whose biochemical functions are so intertwined that understanding any one of them in isolation misses the most important clinical story. The examination in each cluster is mechanistic: what do these nutrients do, at the biochemical level, and what are the cascade consequences when any of them is absent or insufficient? It is historical: what does the clinical record of deficiency disease tell us, and what does that record suggest about the subclinical equivalents that modern populations carry without knowing? And it is clinical: what does the evidence suggest about the tests that reveal what standard medicine cannot see, the foods and interventions that address upstream causes, and the interdependencies between nutrients that mean no single musician can be understood alone?

The book does not ask you to abandon your physician or reject pharmaceutical medicine. It asks you to add a layer of inquiry that the medical system has not been designed to provide: an upstream investigation of the nutritional conditions under which your biology is operating. It asks the question that Goldberger asked of pellagra, that Eijkman asked of beriberi, that Lind asked of scurvy, that Pauling asked of cardiovascular disease, that

Lonsdale asked of dysautonomia, that Hoffer asked of schizophrenia — the question that the institution resisted in every case, that was eventually vindicated in every case, and that remains, a century later, structurally absent from the clinical encounter: not what is wrong, but why.

Two ways to read what follows. Each of the fourteen clusters introduces its nutrients in plain terms under *Meet the Cast* and closes with *The Questions Worth Asking* — the tests and questions worth bringing to a clinician. For a faster read, take a chapter's opening alongside those two, and you have its argument without the biochemistry: what the cluster does, how its failure shows up in a real body, and what to ask.

To go deeper, read the mechanism in between, which goes furthest in the shaded *For the Clinically Curious* boxes — self-contained, so read every one or skip every one, and the argument holds. The book works either way: quickly, for the argument, or slowly, for the machinery.

XII. The Map and the Territory

There is a famous observation in philosophy that the map is not the territory. The map is a representation of the territory, useful for navigation, inevitably incomplete, and dangerous when mistaken for the thing it represents. Modern medicine has a magnificent map. It is drawn in the language of molecular biology, diagnostic imaging, randomized controlled trials, and evidence-based guidelines. It has more resolution in more areas than any map medicine has ever had. It saves lives daily that would otherwise be lost.

But it is still a map, and the territory it was designed to represent is disease — specific, named, categorized, coded. The territory it was not designed to represent — the long pre-clinical period of nutritional depletion, metabolic drift, and systemic deterioration that precedes disease — is mostly blank on the map. Not because it does not exist, but because the cartographers were not asked to survey it.

Margaret, our patient from the opening of this chapter, is living in the unmapped territory. Her five diagnoses represent five points where her deteriorating nutritional and metabolic terrain finally produced pathology visible enough for the map to record. The terrain itself — the energy machinery running without adequate fuel (Cluster 1), the gut gateway damaged by four courses of antibiotics and three years of acid suppression and never restored (Cluster 2), the microbiome quietly reshaped and the immune education it provides quietly withdrawn (Cluster 3), the antioxidant network with gaps that are allowing oxidative damage to accumulate in her arterial walls (Cluster 4), the collagen architecture signaling its distress in bleeding gums and cardiovascular risk (Cluster 5), the hormonal system impaired at the thyroid conversion step and at the adrenal-cortisol interface simultaneously (Cluster 6), the neurological chemistry producing her anxiety from a substrate whose methylation, omega-3 architecture, and GABA cofactors have never been assessed (Clusters 7 and 9), the immune calibration drifting toward the autoimmune permissiveness that is sustaining her Hashimoto's (Cluster 8), and the cascade of protective biological inputs that her diet had quietly eliminated across the six clusters beyond (Clusters 9 through 14) — is not on the map. Nobody gave Margaret a map of the territory. Nobody told her she was living in it.

This book is an attempt to sketch some of that unmapped territory. Not comprehensively — the territory is vast — but in enough depth, for enough of its most important features, that the reader emerges with a different way of asking questions about their health and about the health of people they care for. Not a different set of answers to the questions medicine already asks. A different set of questions.

> *The history of medicine is, among other things, a history of discoveries that were resisted by the institutions that should have embraced them, validated by the passage of time, and incorporated into practice decades later than the evidence warranted. This book describes that pattern. It does not ask you to distrust medicine. It asks you to notice that the pattern has not stopped repeating — and to ask what it might mean for the patients sitting in today's waiting rooms, carrying diagnoses that tomorrow's medicine may recognize as the downstream consequences of upstream causes that nobody thought to look for.*

The fourteen clusters that follow are about specific nutrient systems. They are also about a single argument: that the body's sixty essential non-caloric nutrients are not supplements, not optional additions to a baseline of adequate nutrition, not the province of alternative medicine and health food stores. They are the molecular infrastructure of biological function, the upstream determinants of metabolic health, and the missing variable in the diagnostic equation that produces patients like Margaret: sick, spent, and — in the absence of the questions this book asks — praying.

Standing on the Shoulders of Giants

The Brilliant Minds Who Found Pieces of the Puzzle — and the Complete Picture None of Them Could See Alone

---

"If I have seen further, it is by standing on the shoulders of giants."

— Isaac Newton, 1675

There is a particular kind of intellectual courage required to tell medicine it is wrong. Not wrong about a procedure, or a dosage, or a protocol — but wrong at the level of its most fundamental assumptions about what causes disease and where healing begins.

The men and women discussed in this chapter had that courage. They spent careers — in some cases, entire lifetimes — arguing from evidence that nutritional insufficiency lay upstream of diseases medicine was busy naming, categorizing, and treating downstream. They were largely ignored. Some were ridiculed. Several died before the vindication their work deserved.

This chapter honors them. And it also asks a harder question: if these brilliant, dedicated scientists could each find a piece of the puzzle, why did none of them assemble the complete picture? And what does that incompleteness tell us about how deep the blind spot in modern medicine truly runs?

Derrick Lonsdale and the Thiamine Revolution

Dr. Derrick Lonsdale spent more than five decades arguing a case that mainstream medicine found inconvenient: that thiamine — vitamin B1 — was far more critically depleted in modern populations than anyone acknowledged, and that its insufficiency sat at the root of a staggering range of neurological, cardiac, and metabolic conditions being treated as primary diseases.

His central argument was elegant and mechanistically precise. Thiamine pyrophosphate is an absolute requirement for pyruvate dehydrogenase — the enzyme complex that converts pyruvate into acetyl-CoA, the molecule that enters the Krebs cycle and initiates the production of the electron carriers that drive ATP synthesis. Without thiamine, this gateway is closed. Pyruvate cannot enter the Krebs cycle. It accumulates instead as lactate. The entire downstream energy cascade — from Krebs cycle to electron transport chain to ATP synthase — is starved at its entrance.

Lonsdale understood what medicine consistently refused to accept: that a single nutritional insufficiency, operating at a precise biochemical chokepoint, could produce multi-system disease that looked nothing like a simple vitamin deficiency and everything like a collection of serious named conditions.

He documented cases of dysautonomia, heart failure, neurological deterioration, and metabolic dysfunction that responded — sometimes dramatically — to thiamine supplementation after years of fruitless conventional treatment. He wrote prolifically, collaborated with researchers globally, and constructed a body of evidence that was methodologically rigorous and clinically compelling.

Medicine, for the most part, did not listen.

The reasons are familiar from every cluster in this book. Thiamine deficiency was considered a disease of the past — beriberi, the historic scourge of polished-rice populations, long since conquered. The idea that subclinical thiamine insufficiency could be widespread in modern Western populations, producing disease without the classical presentation of beriberi, sat outside the diagnostic imagination of a profession trained to recognize overt deficiency or nothing at all.

Lonsdale's work represents one of the most important and most neglected bodies of nutritional medicine research of the twentieth century. This book stands firmly on his shoulders.

But here is the striking thing — the observation that opens a door Lonsdale himself may not have fully walked through.

The Missed Parallel: Copper at Complex IV

Lonsdale identified thiamine's role at the entry point of the ATP production cascade — the gateway from glycolysis into the Krebs cycle. His entire life's work rested on the understanding that blocking this single step could produce catastrophic, multi-system energy failure.

He was absolutely right.

What appears to have gone largely unrecognized — even by Lonsdale — is that the ATP production cascade has another nutrient dependency equally critical, equally absolute, and equally invisible to standard medicine. Not at the entry point, but at the final step.

Copper.

Cytochrome c oxidase — Complex IV of the electron transport chain — is the enzyme that accepts electrons from cytochrome c and transfers them to molecular oxygen, reducing it to water. This final reaction is what collapses the electrochemical gradient that drives ATP synthase. Without it, the entire upstream machinery — the Krebs cycle Lonsdale championed, the electron carriers it produces, the protein complexes that transfer them — has nowhere to deliver its output. The chain backs up. ATP synthesis halts. Electrons leak and generate the most destructive free radicals known to biology.

Copper is not a cofactor for Complex IV. *Copper is Complex IV.* Two copper atoms — CuA and CuB — are structurally embedded at the enzyme's active site. They are the chemistry that makes the final reaction chemically possible. There is no workaround, no alternative pathway, no compensatory mechanism. Without copper, the electron transport chain cannot complete its function.

> *Thiamine closes the gate at the entrance of the Krebs cycle. Copper closes the gate at the exit of the electron transport chain. Block either one, and the result is the same: ATP production collapses and the cell starves for energy regardless of how much food the person consumes.*

The symptomatic consequences are strikingly parallel. Both deficiencies produce neurological deterioration — peripheral neuropathy, spinal cord damage, cognitive decline. Both produce cardiac vulnerability. Both generate profound, treatment-resistant fatigue. Both are virtually untested in standard clinical practice. Both mimic serious named conditions that receive diagnoses and treatments that never address the upstream cause.

The comparison deserves to be seen in full:

	Thiamine (B1) — Lonsdale's Focus	Copper — The Missing Parallel
ATP pathway location	Pyruvate → Acetyl-CoA (Krebs cycle entry)	Complex IV — final ETC step
Dependent enzyme	Pyruvate dehydrogenase complex	Cytochrome c oxidase
What fails without it	Krebs cycle cannot be entered	Electron chain cannot complete
Effect on ATP	Production collapses at input	Production collapses at output
Secondary damage	Lactate accumulation, neurological crisis	ROS surge, oxidative catastrophe
Neurological impact	Wernicke's encephalopathy, neuropathy	Myelopathy, peripheral neuropathy
Cardiac impact	Wet beriberi, heart failure	Cardiomyopathy, arterial weakness
Historical disease anchor	Beriberi — population scale	Menkes disease — rare genetic
Modern depletion drivers	Alcohol, refined carbohydrates	Zinc supplementation,

		processed food
Standard testing	Rarely ordered	Almost never ordered
Functional test	Transketolase activity	SOD activity, RBC copper

This parallel is not coincidental. It is the inevitable consequence of two nutrients occupying critical positions in the same biochemical pathway — one at its entrance, one at its exit — both depleted by modern life, both invisible to standard medicine, both capable of producing identical patterns of catastrophic multi-system disease.

The question this raises is not a criticism of Lonsdale. It is a window into the depth of the problem this book addresses.

If one of the twentieth century's most sophisticated nutritional thinkers — a man who spent decades proving that a single nutrient could sit at the upstream root of diseases medicine treated as primary — did not fully articulate copper's equally critical role in the same pathway, what does that tell us about the scale of what conventional medicine, trained to look nowhere near this territory, is missing?

Why Brilliant Minds Found Pieces, Not the Whole

Understanding why even the most insightful nutritional researchers of the past century found pieces of the puzzle without assembling the complete picture is not an academic exercise. It is essential to understanding why this book is necessary — and what it is attempting to do that has not been done before.

The Specialization Trap

Lonsdale went deep on thiamine because depth was required to make the case. The same was true of Pauling on vitamin C, Hoffer on niacin, Price on fat-soluble vitamins, and Klevay on copper. Each committed to one nutrient or one system with the intensity that landmark science demands. That commitment produced genuine insights — and tunnel vision. When you spend decades proving the centrality of one nutrient, it becomes psychologically and professionally difficult to argue that another deserves equal billing. The specialization that produced depth prevented breadth. Each pioneer found their thread and pulled it heroically, without seeing that all the threads were part of the same fabric.

The Testing Problem

Copper's relationship with inflammation through ceruloplasmin creates a diagnostic fog that thiamine testing does not have. A researcher looking at population copper levels in the twentieth century would have encountered apparently normal serum readings in many patients who were functionally deficient at the cellular level — precisely because inflammation artificially elevates the serum measurement. The tools to see through this fog — RBC copper, superoxide dismutase activity, functional ceruloplasmin assessment — were not widely available or understood during the most active years of nutritional medicine research.

Lonsdale had access to transketolase activity testing — a functional measure of thiamine status that cut through the noise. The equivalent functional testing for copper was not comparably established. The deficiency was harder to demonstrate, which made the argument harder to make.

The historical anchor problem compounded this. Thiamine had beriberi, vitamin C had scurvy, niacin had pellagra — dramatic population-scale precedents that gave each researcher a narrative platform for arguing that modern subclinical insufficiency was producing similar if less dramatic consequences. Copper's closest equivalent is Menkes disease: a rare, genetic, pediatric condition that powerfully demonstrates what profound copper deficiency does to the developing body, but a poor platform for arguing that adult dietary insufficiency is widespread and driving common chronic disease. The historical anchor was available but mismatched to the argument that needed to be made.

The Zinc Supplement Epidemic

The widespread zinc supplementation that actively depletes copper through competitive inhibition of intestinal metallothionein is a relatively recent phenomenon, driven by the explosion of the consumer supplement industry in the late twentieth and early twenty-first centuries. The copper-depleting effect of mass zinc consumption may have been far less clinically apparent during the years when most nutritional medicine pioneers were conducting their most active research. The perfect storm of copper depletion we face today — processed diet plus gut dysfunction plus widespread zinc supplementation plus soil mineral depletion — had not fully assembled itself.

The Other Giants

Lonsdale is not alone in this story. The history of nutritional medicine is populated with researchers who each found a critical piece of the puzzle and argued for it courageously against institutional resistance. Understanding what each contributed — and what each missed — illuminates both the importance of their work and the necessity of this book.

Linus Pauling — The Orthomolecular Vision

Linus Pauling — twice, Nobel laureate — argued that the optimal concentration of naturally occurring molecules in the body, particularly vitamins, was the foundation of health. His work on vitamin C was pioneering: he understood that the RDA represented the floor for preventing overt deficiency, not the ceiling for optimal function, and that humans required dramatically higher concentrations for true physiological optimization.

His insight that medicine had defined adequacy far too low — that "not deficient" and "optimally supplied" were entirely different things — is one of the most important intellectual contributions to nutritional medicine. This book's entire argument about the gap between RDA and optimal function rests on Pauling's foundation.

What Pauling's vitamin C focus could not capture was the network nature of nutritional insufficiency. Vitamin C does not operate in isolation. It regenerates vitamin E. It depends on adequate glutathione. It supports carnitine synthesis, which requires iron and niacin alongside it. The single-nutrient focus, however brilliant, could not see the web. Warburg pointed toward the deeper truth that Pauling's single-nutrient focus could not fully reach. Otto Warburg — the German biochemist who won the Nobel Prize in 1931 for discovering the oxygen-transferring enzyme of cellular respiration — had already glimpsed it. His observation that cancer cells abandon the normal aerobic energy metabolism of healthy cells, preferring instead the far less efficient anaerobic pathway even in the presence of oxygen, implied something profound about mitochondrial function: that its failure was not merely an energy problem but a signal of broader cellular breakdown. The Warburg effect, as it became known, is now understood as a consequence of mitochondrial dysfunction — precisely the dysfunction that nutritional insufficiency in the energy cluster produces. Warburg described the endpoint. The nutrients in Cluster 1 govern whether the mitochondria reach it.

Emanuel Cheraskin, a physician and researcher who worked alongside Pauling in the orthomolecular tradition, extended the same argument into clinical language. His concept of the "optimum" — the nutrient intake associated not with the mere absence of deficiency disease but with peak physiological function — gave clinicians a vocabulary for what Pauling had argued biochemically. Together, Pauling and Cheraskin articulated a principle this book treats as foundational: that the RDA marks the floor of a range, not its ceiling, and that the gap between the two is where most of modern chronic disease quietly lives.

Abram Hoffer — The Niacin Pioneer

Dr. Abram Hoffer spent decades demonstrating that high-dose niacin — vitamin B3 — could treat schizophrenia and other psychiatric conditions that medicine was managing with antipsychotic medications producing severe side effects. His work on orthomolecular psychiatry was methodologically careful and clinically documented. It was largely dismissed.

Hoffer understood that NAD+ — the active form derived from niacin — was not merely a vitamin but a fundamental currency of cellular energy and DNA repair. His intuition that depleting this currency could produce psychiatric disease was correct. What his niacin focus could not fully illuminate was that NAD+ depletion was one expression of a broader collapse in the nutritional substrates required for neuronal energy production — a collapse that implicated thiamine, copper, magnesium, and a dozen other nutrients alongside niacin.

Weston A. Price — The Dietary Anthropologist

Dr. Weston A. Price traveled the world in the 1930s studying the health of traditional populations eating indigenous diets and comparing them to populations that had adopted industrialized Western food. His photographic and biochemical documentation of the physical degeneration that followed dietary industrialization remains one of the most compelling empirical arguments ever assembled for the nutritional root of modern chronic disease.

Price identified fat-soluble vitamins — what he called "activator X" (now understood to be vitamin K2), along with vitamins A and D — as critical missing factors in industrialized diets. He understood that the physical structure of the body, from dental arch formation to skeletal development, depended on nutritional inputs that industrialized food systematically stripped away.

His framework was visual and anthropological rather than biochemical and mechanistic. It could not drill down to the mitochondrial level — to Complex IV and cytochrome c oxidase — where the molecular consequences of nutritional insufficiency ultimately play out. The picture was vast and correct in its broad strokes, but lacked the molecular resolution that the intervening decades of biochemical research have made possible.

Leslie Klevay — The Copper Cardiovascular Pioneer

Dr. Leslie Klevay deserves special mention in a book that places copper at the center of its argument. His research over several decades built the case that copper deficiency was a significant and underrecognized contributor to cardiovascular disease — documenting the effects of copper insufficiency on lipid profiles, cardiac function, and arterial wall integrity with careful experimental methodology.

Klevay was right. His cardiovascular work stands. But even his copper focus was narrower than the full picture this book assembles. The connection from copper to Complex IV, to the complete collapse of ATP production, to the multi-system disease cascade that follows — the neurological, immunological, structural, and metabolic dimensions of copper insufficiency — was not the center of his argument. He found the cardiovascular thread and pulled it. The full tapestry remained unassembled.

Bruce Ames — The Triage Theory

Dr. Bruce Ames, biochemist at UC Berkeley, proposed what may be the most intellectually elegant framework in nutritional medicine: the triage theory. When micronutrients are scarce, the body prioritizes their use for immediate survival — acute functions like blood clotting, muscle contraction, and immune response — at the expense of long-term maintenance functions like DNA repair, mitochondrial integrity, and cellular resilience.

The result, Ames argued, is that subclinical micronutrient insufficiency — insufficient to produce obvious deficiency disease — accelerates aging, increases cancer risk, and drives the accumulation of cellular damage that expresses itself as chronic disease decades later. The body survives in the short term while quietly degrading in the long term, and standard medicine, focused on acute disease, never sees the slow catastrophe accumulating beneath.

Ames's triage theory is perhaps the closest existing framework to the argument this book makes. But it remains primarily a theoretical framework — elegant and important, but not yet translated into the comprehensive clinical mapping of 60 essential nutrients, their specific insufficiency disease connections, and the testing and restoration protocols that would make it actionable for the practicing physician or the suffering patient.

Roger Williams — The Biochemistry of the Individual

Roger Williams was a biochemist at the University of Texas whose 1956 book Biochemical Individuality proposed something that should have been obvious but was not: that human beings vary dramatically in their nutritional requirements, and that this variation is not pathological but normal. The Recommended Dietary Allowance — established by the nutrition establishment in the 1940s — represented a population average. Williams demonstrated that the distribution of human nutritional requirements around that average was wide, not narrow. The person who needs three times the average intake of a given nutrient to maintain optimal enzymatic function will not be flagged as deficient by any standard test. They will simply be sick, and their physician will look everywhere except where Williams pointed.

Williams also understood something the other giants only partially grasped: that nutrients do not act in isolation. They function in networks — interdependent, mutually regulating, collectively determining the biochemical environment in which every cell operates. He called this the "teamwork" of nutrients — a concept that anticipated by decades the systems-biology thinking that the cluster architecture of this book now makes structural. Where every other pioneer in this chapter pulled one thread, Williams described the fabric.

Why was Williams ignored? For the same structural reasons every pioneer in this chapter was ignored — and for one additional reason unique to his contribution. Biochemical individuality, taken seriously, requires medicine to treat every patient as a distinct biochemical entity requiring personalized nutritional assessment. It cannot be reduced to a population guideline, a standard protocol, or a reimbursable panel. It is, by its nature, the opposite of standardization. And standardization is what medicine runs on.

His insight is indispensable to this book. Every cluster that follows is built on the understanding that there is no single correct dose of any nutrient, no universal optimal blood level, no one-size protocol that serves every patient equally. What the clusters describe are the systems and their nutritional requirements. What Williams established is that the margin between adequacy and insufficiency differs for every person within those systems — shaped by genetics, by stress, and by the accumulation of depletions that a lifetime in the modern world reliably produces.

The Wider Lineage

The lineage extends further than any single chapter can hold. Christiaan Eijkman traced beriberi to polished rice a full generation before Lonsdale would spend his career on the same vitamin, proving as early as 1897 that a disease assumed to be infectious was, in fact, nutritional — a pattern this book has now traced across a century and sixty nutrients.

Denis Burkitt, comparing colorectal cancer rates between Connecticut and rural Africa, found a tenfold difference and pointed to fiber and gut transit time as the explanation — one of the earliest demonstrations that comparing populations, not just individuals, could reveal a dietary cause hiding in plain sight.

George and Mildred Burr identified the essential fatty acids in the 1930s, work for which Mildred has gone largely uncredited despite being equally responsible for the discovery.

And Andrew Saul, decades later, did not discover a new mechanism — he built the bridge between everything these researchers found and the patients who needed to know it, founding the Orthomolecular Medicine News Service and making fifty years of buried science freely available to anyone willing to read.

Each of them, in their own register, asked the same upstream question this book asks. None of them are forgotten here.

What This Book Does Differently

This book does not claim to supersede the work of Lonsdale, Pauling, Hoffer, Price, Klevay, Williams or Ames. Their contributions are foundational, and this book would be impossible without them. What it claims — and what the evidence supports — is that assembling their insights into a unified framework reveals something none of them, working in their individual disciplines, could fully see.

> *Each pioneer found their thread and pulled it heroically. This book looks at the loom.*

The unified framework this book proposes is this: modern chronic disease is not a collection of separate conditions requiring separate treatments. It is largely the downstream consequence of simultaneous insufficiency across the 60 essential non-caloric nutrients — vitamins, minerals, trace elements, amino acids, and biochemical cofactors — that power every cellular function in the human body.

The unified framework is expressed in fourteen clusters. Each cluster groups the nutrients that govern a specific biological system — not because the grouping is convenient but because the biology demands it. What follows is a map of the territory the reader is about to enter.

Cluster 1: The Energy Architects. Twelve nutrients — including the B vitamins, magnesium, iron, copper, CoQ10, carnitine, and PQQ — collectively operate the three-stage machinery of cellular energy production. When any of them is insufficient, every high-energy tissue in the body degrades simultaneously: the brain, the heart, the immune system, the gut wall. The fatigue that medicine calls idiopathic, the dysautonomia that goes undiagnosed for years, the heart failure that worsens on the medication prescribed to treat it — these are energy stories. Cluster 1 identifies the twelve musicians without whom the concert cannot begin.

Cluster 2: The Master Gateway. The gut wall — one cell thick, spanning a surface area the size of a tennis court — is the gateway through which every nutrient in every other cluster must pass before it can reach the cells that need it. Ten nutrients maintain this gateway: glutamine, zinc, vitamins D and A, butyrate, threonine, glycine, omega-3 fatty acids, vitamin C, and phosphatidylcholine. When the gateway is compromised, every downstream intervention works at a fraction of its potential. This is the prerequisite cluster. It comes second because it must.

Cluster 3: The Garden Within. The 38 trillion microbial cells inhabiting the gut constitute an ecosystem as consequential as any organ in the body. They synthesize vitamins, convert dietary compounds into their bioactive forms, program regulatory immune circuits, produce ninety percent of the body's serotonin, and determine whether the nutrients consumed reach the cells that need them. Cluster 3 examines the dietary inputs, bacterial species, and microbial metabolites — particularly short-chain fatty acids and the tryptophan-serotonin-kynurenine axis — that determine whether this ecosystem supports health or quietly undermines it. The depression, the autoimmunity, the metabolic syndrome: many of these are microbiome stories that medicine has labeled without ever looking at the garden.

Cluster 4: The Antioxidant Shield. Every cell burns fuel and in doing so generates fire. Eight nutrients — selenium, vitamins C and E, copper, zinc, manganese, glutathione, and alpha-lipoic acid — form a cascading network that contains that fire. The network is interdependent in a precise sequence: vitamin E neutralizes the radical in the membrane, vitamin C regenerates vitamin E, glutathione regenerates vitamin C, riboflavin and niacin regenerate glutathione, and alpha-lipoic acid can reset the entire cascade simultaneously. Remove any link and the fire spreads further before being contained. The oxidative damage that medicine has labeled as aging, cancer initiation, cardiovascular disease, and neurodegeneration is largely the accumulated consequence of a shield with holes.

Cluster 5: The Structural Architects. Collagen is the most abundant protein in the body, forming the scaffolding of bone, tendon, ligament, arterial wall, and skin. Its synthesis and maturation requires eleven nutrients working in precise sequence: vitamin A to express the collagen gene, vitamin C and iron to complete the protein chain, copper to cross-link the fibers into their load-bearing form, glycine and proline as structural amino acids, vitamin K2 to route calcium into the matrix rather than arterial walls, and manganese, silicon, zinc, and phosphorus for the surrounding ground substance. Osteoporosis, arterial fragility, slow wound healing, and bleeding gums are not separate conditions.

They are different expressions of a single structural insufficiency that medicine has never assembled into one story.

Cluster 6: The Hormonal Regulators. The thyroid axis alone requires five nutrients to synthesize its hormones, a sixth to convert them to their active form, and a seventh for the receptor through which they signal. The adrenal glands concentrate vitamin C at higher levels than any other tissue and consume it continuously during stress. The insulin receptor requires magnesium to phosphorylate its downstream cascade. Potassium maintains the membrane voltage without which every hormone signal fails to propagate. The patient who remains hypothyroid on adequate medication, the person whose insulin resistance worsens on a calorie-restricted diet, the individual whose adrenal system has collapsed under chronic stress — these are nutritional stories told in the language of endocrinology.

Cluster 7: The Neurological Foundations. Every neurotransmitter the brain produces is synthesized through a biochemical pathway that requires specific nutritional cofactors. Serotonin requires iron and B6. Dopamine requires iron, B6, copper, and vitamin C in sequence. GABA requires B6 to be converted from glutamate — its absence tilts the brain toward excitation. Twelve nutrients govern the neurological foundations: the B vitamins for neurotransmitter synthesis and myelin maintenance, DHA for the membrane architecture through which every signal travels, zinc and magnesium for the receptor dynamics that determine whether signals are transmitted or lost, iron and vitamin D for the developmental and regulatory functions that persist throughout life. The partial response to antidepressants, the anxiety that medication contains but never resolves, the cognitive decline that accelerates with age — these are neurological chemistry stories whose upstream chapters have never been read.

Cluster 8: The Immune Architects. The immune system does not fail at random. It fails because it was not given what it needed to build, calibrate, and restrain itself. Ten nutrients — vitamin D, zinc, selenium, vitamins A and C, iron, omega-3 EPA, magnesium, glutamine, and glycine — determine whether the immune system mounts an adequate defense, resolves inflammation when the threat is eliminated, and maintains the regulatory tolerance that prevents it from attacking the body's own tissues. The autoimmune epidemic — rheumatoid arthritis, Hashimoto's, lupus, multiple sclerosis — is substantially an immune calibration story. The 2022 discovery that magnesium is required for T-cell cytotoxic function against cancer cells is one of many examples of how close the relationship between nutritional status and immune competence truly is.

Cluster 9: The Methylation Network. Methylation is the body's master control dial — the molecular mechanism by which gene expression is continuously regulated, neurotransmitters are inactivated, homocysteine is cleared, and the substrates for phospholipid and creatine synthesis are produced. Eight nutrients drive this cycle: folate, B12, B6, riboflavin, choline, betaine, zinc, and magnesium. The MTHFR gene variant — carried by approximately forty percent of the population in some form — is not a genetic sentence. It is a nutritional requirement: a narrowed margin for these eight nutrients whose clinical expression is determined entirely by whether that narrowed margin is met. Elevated homocysteine, treatment-resistant depression, recurrent pregnancy loss, accelerated epigenetic aging — these are methylation stories whose upstream cause is assessable with an inexpensive blood panel that is almost never ordered.

Cluster 10: The Detoxification Network. The liver processes every molecule that enters the bloodstream — medications, environmental toxins, hormones, metabolic byproducts — through a two-phase system. Phase I activates toxins for processing; Phase II conjugates them for excretion. Both phases depend entirely on nutritional cofactors: glutathione, glycine, taurine, sulfur amino acids, and the B vitamins, among others. When Phase I is active, but Phase II is nutrient-depleted, reactive intermediates accumulate and cause more damage than the original compound. The chemical sensitivity, the hormone imbalance driven by impaired estrogen clearance, the toxin accumulation that worsens every other system — these are detoxification stories. Cluster 10 maps the network and explains why stimulating detoxification without nutritional support for its completion is worse than not stimulating it at all.

Cluster 11: The Amino Acid Foundation. Protein is not a single nutrient. It is a delivery vehicle for thirteen amino acids — nine essential, four conditionally essential — each of which has specific and irreplaceable roles. Tryptophan is the sole precursor for serotonin and melatonin. Tyrosine and phenylalanine are the backbone of the entire catecholamine cascade. Glycine is the rate-limiting amino acid for collagen synthesis and glutathione production simultaneously. Glutamine fuels both the gut lining and the rapidly dividing immune cells that defend it. The question is not simply how much protein — it is which amino acids, from which sources, absorbed through a gut that may be functioning at a fraction of its capacity. The muscle wasting of aging, the mood disorder that does not respond to medication, the poor wound healing that persists despite adequate nutrition — these are amino acid stories.

Cluster 12: The Fat-Soluble Foundations. Vitamins A, D, E, and K are fat-soluble — and they were removed from the food supply by the low-fat dietary era as efficiently as if they had been deliberately extracted. Vitamin A is the master regulator of cell differentiation. Vitamin D is a steroid hormone governing over 2,000 genes across virtually every tissue type. Vitamin E is the membrane antioxidant that protects the polyunsaturated fats in cell walls from oxidative destruction. Vitamin K2 is the calcium traffic director — routing it into bone and away from arterial walls. Phospholipids provide the membrane scaffold on which all four vitamins depend for absorption and function. These vitamins are not independent. They share nuclear receptors, compete for the same transport proteins, and depend on each other for full function. The fat-phobic dietary advice of the past half-century produced a population deficient in all four simultaneously.

Cluster 13: The Essential Fatty Acids. Between 1960 and 2000, the Western food supply replaced traditional animal fats with industrially produced seed oils, shifting the dietary omega-3 to omega-6 ratio from an ancestral 1:4 to the modern 1:15 to 1:20. This was not a minor dietary adjustment. It was a wholesale change in the fat composition of every cell membrane in the body — including the neuronal membranes through which every thought and mood is processed, the immune cell membranes through which every inflammatory response is initiated or resolved, and the arterial membranes whose prostaglandin balance determines whether the cardiovascular system remains elastic or begins to stiffen. DHA alone constitutes sixty percent of the brain's structural fat. The epidemic of depression, the chronic inflammation underlying cardiovascular disease, the failure of immunity to resolve — these are fatty acid stories. Cluster 13 describes the accidental experiment nobody designed, nobody monitored, and nobody has yet fully reckoned with.

Cluster 14: The Supporting Cast — Protective Compounds. Modern food processing did not merely reduce vitamin and mineral content. It eliminated entire categories of biological compounds that traditional diets had always delivered — compounds whose absence medicine has never thought to measure, whose roles it has never thought to investigate, and whose loss it has never thought to name. Sulforaphane, quercetin, curcumin, resveratrol, lutein, zeaxanthin, spermidine, inositol — these are not fringe supplements. They are the signal shapers, the tissue guardians, the cellular housekeeping crew that activates the body's own cytoprotective gene expression, maintains the visual system, clears damaged cellular machinery through autophagy, and modulates the inflammatory and detoxification networks that every other cluster depends upon. Their absence does not produce a named deficiency syndrome. It produces something subtler and more pervasive: a slow failure of the body's own protective systems, accumulating silently over decades before it becomes a condition anyone thinks to diagnose. Cluster 14 names what was eliminated, explains what it did, and asks why its absence has never appeared on a single laboratory requisition form.

These fourteen clusters do not tell fourteen separate stories. They tell one story, from fourteen angles. The energy architects cannot function if the gut gateway does not absorb their nutrients. The antioxidant shield cannot be maintained if the methylation network cannot regenerate glutathione. The immune system cannot calibrate itself without the microbiome that educated it. The structural scaffolding degrades faster when the hormonal system is impaired. Every cluster depends on every other cluster in ways that become visible only when all fourteen are held in view simultaneously. That is what this book does. That is what has not been done before at this scale.

The Systemic Reason the Picture Stayed Incomplete

The incompleteness of these pioneers' work was not a limitation of individual vision. It was systemic — and the system has not changed. These researchers published in peer-reviewed journals, presented at conferences, and made their cases in full view of the medical establishment. The establishment chose, consistently and institutionally, not to integrate their work. The reasons are structural, not accidental:

- **Medical training allocates minimal time to clinical nutrition.** A physician completing a standard medical degree in the United States receives, on average, fewer than 25 hours of nutrition education across four years of training. Trace mineral biochemistry — the territory where Lonsdale, Klevay, and their peers were working — is largely absent from this thin curriculum.
- **The pharmaceutical model defines the research agenda.** Nutrients cannot be patented. A mineral found in food cannot generate the return on investment that justifies the billions required to move a novel pharmaceutical compound through clinical trials and regulatory approval. The research

infrastructure of modern medicine is built on patentable interventions. Nutritional insufficiency, however well documented, generates no revenue stream and attracts no institutional investment.

- **The silo structure of medical specialization prevents synthesis.** A cardiologist treating heart failure does not communicate with the neurologist treating the same patient's peripheral neuropathy, who does not communicate with the rheumatologist treating their osteoporosis, who does not communicate with the hematologist investigating their treatment-resistant anemia. Each specialist treats their slice perfectly. No one looks at the whole. And the whole — the pattern that would reveal a common upstream nutritional root — is never assembled.
- **Standard laboratory panels do not test for nutritional insufficiency.** The tests that would reveal what the pioneers were arguing — RBC magnesium, RBC copper, superoxide dismutase activity, transketolase activity, functional B12, selenium status — are not on routine panels. A physician must actively suspect a nutritional root cause and specifically order these tests. That conscious step never happens in a system where the training never planted the seed.

This is not a conspiracy. There is no coordinated suppression of nutritional medicine. What there is, instead, is a system that evolved around pharmacological intervention, that trains physicians in the language of disease management rather than root cause investigation, and that has built its research, reimbursement, and institutional structures around an approach to medicine that makes nutritional insufficiency literally invisible.

The pioneers discussed in this chapter worked against that system with extraordinary dedication. They were not wrong. They were incomplete — because no individual working in the specialization-driven, institutionally resistant landscape of twentieth-century medicine could be anything else.

This Book as Completion, Not Contradiction

Every cluster that follows in this book is built on the foundations these pioneers laid. Lonsdale's thiamine work informs Cluster 1 on the energy architects and the ATP gateway. Pauling's orthomolecular framework informs the argument that RDA represents a floor, not an optimum. Hoffer's niacin research informs the NAD+ story woven through Clusters 1 and 7. Price's anthropological documentation informs Clusters 12 and 13 on fat-soluble vitamins and essential fatty acids. Klevay's copper cardiovascular work informs both Cluster 1 (where copper completes the electron transport chain) and Cluster 5 (where it cross-links collagen). Ames's triage theory informs the framework throughout for understanding how subclinical insufficiency accumulates into catastrophic disease.

What this book adds is the synthesis. The 60-nutrient landscape mapped in its entirety. The converging mechanisms — energy failure, oxidative stress, structural degradation, gut barrier failure, microbiome disruption, methylation impairment, hormonal dysregulation, neurological insufficiency, immune miscalibration, and more — identified and mapped through fourteen clusters to show how nutritional insufficiency produces the full spectrum of modern chronic disease. The testing framework that makes the invisible visible. The clinical road map that translates biochemical understanding into actionable patient care.

And the systemic argument that none of them could make with sufficient force: that this is not a collection of individual nutrient stories. It is a unified theory of chronic disease rooted in nutritional insufficiency and enabled by a medical system structurally designed to miss it.

> *Lonsdale found that thiamine deficiency silenced one musician at the entrance of the energy orchestra. This book shows that sixty musicians play simultaneously in fourteen sections — and that modern life, modern medicine, and modern food have left most of the seats empty. No single musician tells the story. The silence of the orchestra does.*

The giants whose work precedes this book were not wrong. They were looking through straws at a landscape that required a panorama. They were brilliant scientists working heroically within the constraints of their time, their discipline, and the institutional resistance they faced.

This book is not standing against them. It is standing on them — as high as their shoulders will allow — and finally looking at the whole.

---

* * *

The fourteen clusters that follow will take you through the sixty essential non-caloric nutrients, grouped by the systems they collectively govern — their biochemical roles, their depletion pathways, the diseases their combined insufficiency produces, and the tests that reveal what standard medicine cannot see. Each cluster is a section of the orchestra. This introduction has shown you what the complete performance sounds like when the musicians are missing.

By the time you reach the final pages, the picture that no individual pioneer could assemble will be complete. And you will understand — with clarity that standard medicine does not yet possess — why so many people are sick, spent, and praying for answers that their doctors were never trained to find.

Cluster 1

The Energy Architects

How Twelve Nutrients Power Every Cell in Your Body — and What Happens When Even One Goes Missing

"The body does not run on willpower. It runs on chemistry. And chemistry runs on fuel."

I. The Tiredness That Never Lifted

Margaret had been tired for three years. Not the kind of tiredness that a good night's sleep fixes. The kind that lives behind the eyes and in the legs and in that particular flatness of motivation that makes even small decisions feel effortful. She had mentioned it at every annual check-up. The bloods, as her primary care physician put it with reassuring confidence each time, were completely normal. Her thyroid was being managed. Her blood pressure was controlled. There was no obvious reason for the fatigue.

What nobody had checked — what no routine panel in any of her five specialist visits had included — was the status of the twelve nutrients whose collective job is to keep the machinery of cellular energy production running. Thiamine. Riboflavin. Niacin. Pantothenic acid. Magnesium. Iron. Copper. Zinc. Potassium.

Coenzyme Q10. Carnitine. And the less familiar but no less essential: pyrroloquinoline quinone, known as PQQ, the only nutritional compound known to stimulate the formation of entirely new mitochondria.

The mitochondria — those small, ancient, extraordinarily complex structures found in virtually every cell in the human body — are the reason any of this matters. They are where the energy of food is converted into the energy of life. They are where everything the body does, from pumping the heart to firing a synapse to mounting an immune response to repairing a strand of DNA, ultimately gets its power. And they are, in their functioning, entirely dependent on the nutrients this chapter describes.

Margaret's fatigue was not a mystery. It was a signal. The orchestra of her energy metabolism was trying to play, and several of its essential musicians had quietly left the stage.

II. Meet the Cast

Twelve musicians make up the energy orchestra described in this chapter. Each has a name, a role, and a section of the energy cascade it alone can play. They are introduced briefly here so the reader can hold the full ensemble in view before meeting each one in depth.

- **Thiamine (B1)** — The Gatekeeper. Unlocks the entrance to the Krebs cycle. Without it, the concert never begins.
- **Riboflavin (B2)** — The Electron Highway. Carries electrons through Complexes I and II of the energy chain and regenerates the body's master antioxidant.
- **Niacin (B3) and NAD+** — The Energy Currency. The most important electron carrier in the entire cascade, donating electrons at three separate Krebs cycle steps. Also the substrate for DNA repair.
- **Pantothenic Acid (B5)** — The Gate's Key. Builds Coenzyme A, the molecule that carries fuel into the Krebs cycle. No B5, no entry ticket.
- **Magnesium** — The Activation Key. Supports energy enzymes throughout all three stages and — crucially — must bind to every ATP molecule produced before that ATP can be used by anything in the body.
- **Iron** — The Structural Scaffolding. Forms the iron-sulfur clusters and heme groups through which electrons are physically passed between the complexes of the energy chain.
- **Copper** — The Terminal Gate. Embedded in Complex IV — the final step of the energy chain — copper is the chemistry that completes the electron transfer to oxygen. Without it, the entire upstream process backs up and the factory floods with free radicals.
- **Zinc** — The Precision Instrument. Supports glycolytic enzymes and Complex IV structure, and shares an

absorption mechanism with copper whose balance determines the fate of both.

- **Potassium** — The Membrane Voltage. Maintains the electrochemical conditions across the mitochondrial membrane without which ATP synthase — the turbine that produces ATP — cannot spin.
- **Coenzyme Q10** — The Mobile Messenger. The only molecule that can collect electrons from Complexes I and II and deliver them to Complex III. Without CoQ10, the hand-off cannot happen and the chain stalls mid-performance.
- **Carnitine** — The Fat Transporter. Escorts fatty acids across the mitochondrial membrane so they can be burned for fuel. Without carnitine, fat cannot reach the furnace regardless of how much the body carries.
- **PQQ** — The Mitochondrial Architect. The only nutritional compound known to stimulate the formation of entirely new mitochondria. Where every other musician in this chapter improves the performance of the existing orchestra, PQQ recruits new players to join it.

These twelve musicians do not perform in sequence — one finishing before the next begins. They perform simultaneously, in the continuous, overlapping, interdependent way of an orchestra mid-concert. The sections that follow introduce each one in depth. But the cast is named here because the full ensemble must be visible before the individual performances make complete sense.

III. The Orchestra in the Cell

Throughout this book, the sixty essential non-caloric nutrients are understood as musicians in an orchestra. It is not a decorative metaphor. It is a precise one.

A symphony orchestra does not work by each musician playing their part in isolation and the audience hearing the sum. The music emerges from the relationships between instruments — from harmony, from timing, from the way the strings support the brass and the percussion anchors the winds. Remove a single section and the piece does not merely sound incomplete. It sounds wrong in ways that no amount of compensating effort from the remaining musicians can fully correct.

The energy orchestra described in this chapter works exactly this way. Twelve nutrients, each playing a distinct and irreplaceable part. Each dependent on the others for context and function. Remove thiamine and the gateway into the energy cycle closes — no other B vitamin can substitute. Remove magnesium and the ATP molecules produced cannot be activated for use — the energy sits in the cell like locked currency. Remove copper and the final step of electron transport cannot complete — the entire upstream process backs up, and the electrons that were supposed to produce energy instead generate the free radicals that damage everything around them.

Modern medicine, when it investigates fatigue at all, tends to check a single player — thyroid, perhaps, or iron, or occasionally vitamin D. It is looking for a single missing instrument in a twelve-piece ensemble. Finding the thyroid within normal limits, it concludes the orchestra is fine. The music playing in Margaret's cells tells a different story.

> *The body's energy system is not twelve separate functions that happen to occur in the same cell. It is one integrated process, played by twelve musicians simultaneously, in which the performance of each depends on all the others. This is not a metaphor for how nutrients work. It is a description of what actually happens in every mitochondrion in every cell of every person reading this page.*

IV. The Power Station: A Map for the General Reader

Before meeting each musician individually, it helps to understand the concert hall they are playing in. The production of ATP — adenosine triphosphate, the molecule that powers every biological process in the human body — follows a precise sequence through three connected stages. Understanding this sequence is not required to benefit from this book. But understanding it changes how the nutrient depletions that follow feel. They stop being abstract biochemical deficits and become something more visceral: a power station going dark, room by room.

Stage One: Glycolysis — Breaking the Sugar

Every cell begins extracting energy from food in the cytoplasm — the fluid outside the mitochondria — through a process called glycolysis. Glucose, the basic unit of carbohydrate, is broken down in a series of ten chemical steps into a molecule called pyruvate. This stage produces a small but immediate yield: two molecules of ATP per glucose molecule. It also produces electron carriers — NADH — that will be needed later. Glycolysis requires magnesium at multiple steps, and zinc for one of its key enzymes. It is the opening movement of the energy symphony, establishing the theme that the rest of the piece will develop.

Stage Two: The Krebs Cycle — Extracting the Electrons

Pyruvate crosses from the cytoplasm into the mitochondria, where it is converted into a molecule called acetyl-CoA — the entry ticket into the Krebs cycle. This conversion is irreversible and absolute. It requires thiamine as its essential cofactor. No thiamine, no entry. The gate is closed, regardless of how much glucose or how many calories are available.

Inside the Krebs cycle — also called the TCA cycle or citric acid cycle — acetyl-CoA is processed through eight steps that extract electrons from food molecules and load them onto carrier molecules, principally NADH and FADH2. These carriers are not energy themselves. They are the trucks that transport electrons to the real energy production line: the electron transport chain. The Krebs cycle needs thiamine again at one of its internal steps, riboflavin for the FADH2 carriers it produces, niacin for the NADH carriers, magnesium as a cofactor throughout, and manganese for one of its protective enzymes.

Think of the Krebs cycle as a loading dock. Raw materials arrive, get processed, and the valuable cargo — loaded electron carriers — departs for the factory floor.

Stage Three: The Electron Transport Chain — The Factory Floor

The electron transport chain is the most sophisticated molecular machinery in biology, and it is where the overwhelming majority of the body's ATP is produced. Embedded in the inner membrane of each mitochondrion, it consists of four protein complexes — numbered I through IV — that pass electrons down an energy gradient like a bucket brigade, using the released energy to pump hydrogen ions across the membrane and create the electrochemical gradient that drives ATP synthase.

Picture a waterfall. The electrons, loaded onto carriers in the Krebs cycle, arrive at the top. As they tumble through the four complexes, the energy of their descent pumps hydrogen ions into a reservoir. When enough pressure builds, the ions flow back through ATP synthase — a molecular turbine — and their flow generates ATP. This is where the real power is produced. Glycolysis generates two ATP per glucose. The electron transport chain generates approximately thirty-four.

Copper sits at Complex IV — the final complex in the chain, where electrons are transferred to oxygen to form water. This is not a supporting role. Copper atoms are embedded in the enzyme itself and are the chemistry by which the final reaction occurs. Without copper, Complex IV cannot function. The electrons back up. The whole chain stalls. The waterfall stops turning the turbine.

Iron sits throughout the chain in the form of iron-sulfur clusters and heme groups — the molecular scaffolding through which electrons are passed between complexes. CoQ10, produced by the body but requiring adequate nutritional precursors, acts as the mobile electron carrier between complexes — the courier that picks up electrons at Complex I and II and delivers them to Complex III. Without CoQ10, the hand-offs cannot happen.

And at the end — when the ATP has been produced — magnesium performs one final essential service. ATP does not exist in its active form as a free molecule. It exists as a magnesium-ATP complex. Magnesium is the activation key. Without it, the ATP produced by this entire elaborate process cannot be used. The factory has run, the product has been made, and the warehouse door is locked.

> *The human body produces approximately forty kilograms of ATP every day — roughly its own body weight in energy currency. Every milligram of that production passes through the system described above. Every nutrient named in this chapter is not optional equipment. It is load-bearing architecture.*

V. The Musicians, One by One

Each nutrient in this cluster plays a distinct role in the energy orchestra. What follows is not a list of definitions. It is an account of what happens — in the body, in the cells, in the life of a person — when each musician is absent or playing below their best.

Thiamine — The Gatekeeper

Thiamine — vitamin B1 — is the gatekeeper of the entire energy production process. Its active form, thiamine pyrophosphate, is the cofactor that the pyruvate dehydrogenase complex requires to convert pyruvate into acetyl-CoA. There is no substitute. There is no workaround. When thiamine is insufficient, pyruvate cannot enter the Krebs cycle. It backs up and is converted to lactic acid instead. The cells begin running on emergency power — anaerobic glycolysis — generating two ATP where the full process would generate thirty-four.

Thiamine also operates at a second critical junction inside the Krebs cycle itself, where a related enzyme, alpha-ketoglutarate dehydrogenase, requires it. This second checkpoint matters particularly for the brain and nervous system, where alpha-ketoglutarate is a precursor to the neurotransmitters that regulate mood, anxiety, and autonomic function.

The clinical consequences of thiamine insufficiency were described under the name beriberi — a disease that nineteenth-century medicine thought it had solved. The solution was partial. The acute, dramatic beriberi of rice-eating populations was addressed by fortification and public health measures. What was not addressed, and what Derrick Lonsdale spent five decades documenting, was the subclinical thiamine insufficiency of modern populations eating high-carbohydrate diets — a population that does not develop paralytic beriberi but develops something that looks, from a diagnostic distance, like chronic fatigue, dysautonomia, anxiety, irritable bowel syndrome, and cardiac dysfunction. The presentations are different. The upstream cause is the same.

Modern life depletes thiamine through several routes simultaneously. Refined carbohydrates and sugar increase thiamine demand — the more glucose the body metabolizes, the more thiamine it requires. Alcohol actively destroys thiamine in the gut wall. Raw fish contains thiaminase, an enzyme that degrades it. Coffee and tea contain compounds that reduce its absorption. Chronic stress increases demand by accelerating the metabolic rate. And the proton pump inhibitors that Margaret and millions of others take daily reduce stomach acid, impairing thiamine's absorption before it even reaches the bloodstream.

Its essential partner: Magnesium is required to phosphorylate thiamine into its active thiamine pyrophosphate form. A person can consume adequate thiamine and be functionally deficient because insufficient magnesium prevents its activation. This thiamine-magnesium dependency is almost never discussed clinically.

Riboflavin — The Electron Highway

Riboflavin — vitamin B2 — is the origin of two electron carrier molecules that are indispensable to the energy chain: FAD and FMN. FADH2 — the loaded form of FAD — is produced in the Krebs cycle and carries electrons to Complex II of the electron transport chain. FMN is embedded in Complex I itself, the first and largest complex in the chain, where it receives electrons from NADH.

Riboflavin insufficiency therefore creates a bottleneck at two simultaneous points in the energy cascade. The Krebs cycle cannot efficiently generate its electron carriers, and Complex I cannot efficiently receive the electrons that do arrive. The effect is not catastrophic in the way that thiamine deficiency is catastrophic. It is gradual and diffuse — a dimming rather than a shutdown — which is precisely what makes it so easy to miss.

Riboflavin also plays a role that connects the energy orchestra to the antioxidant orchestra: it is required to regenerate glutathione after it has neutralized a free radical. Without adequate riboflavin, the body's master antioxidant cannot complete its recycling cycle. Energy impairment and oxidative stress accumulate together, as they so often do when a single nutrient is depleted — because the same nutrients that power the engine also protect it from the combustion products of its own running.

Its essential partners: Riboflavin works in close coordination with niacin in the electron transport chain — FAD and NAD+ are the two primary electron carriers, and the system requires both.

Riboflavin also supports the MTHFR enzyme in the methylation network, which is why riboflavin status affects the clinical expression of MTHFR gene variants far more than the variants themselves are often acknowledged to do.

Niacin and NAD+ — The Energy Currency

Niacin — vitamin B3 — is the precursor to NAD+ (nicotinamide adenine dinucleotide), the most important electron carrier in cellular energy metabolism. NAD+ accepts electrons at three separate steps in the Krebs cycle to produce NADH, the fully loaded electron carrier that delivers the majority of electrons to the electron transport chain. Of the approximately thirty-four ATP molecules generated from one glucose molecule through the full aerobic pathway, the great majority trace their origin to NADH-donated electrons.

Beyond energy metabolism, NAD+ is the substrate for a family of enzymes called sirtuins — proteins that regulate gene expression, cellular stress response, and longevity — and for PARP enzymes, which repair damaged DNA. NAD+ is, in this sense, both the fuel for the engine and the maintenance budget for the entire cellular factory. When it is depleted, not only does energy production decline but the mechanisms that repair the damage caused by insufficient energy also fail.

NAD+ levels decline with age — a well-documented finding that has generated significant interest in nicotinamide mononucleotide (NMN) and nicotinamide riboside (NR) as precursors that may more efficiently raise intracellular NAD+ than niacin itself. The research here is genuinely promising, though the clinical translation remains evolving. What is not evolving is the evidence that niacin insufficiency — producing the clinical syndrome of pellagra in its frank form, and the subclinical equivalent of cognitive impairment, skin vulnerability, and metabolic dysfunction in its modern form — remains far more prevalent than the medical profession acknowledges.

Dr. Abram Hoffer's decades of clinical work demonstrated that NAD+ depletion extended well beyond energy metabolism into the terrain of psychiatric disease — that schizophrenia, anxiety disorders, and depression had a measurable niacin-NAD+ component that pharmacological management was not addressing. Medicine dismissed Hoffer as an outlier. The biochemistry he was describing has only become more clearly documented in the years since.

Its essential partner: Riboflavin (FAD) and niacin (NAD+) are the two primary electron carrier systems in the chain. They are not interchangeable — they donate electrons to different complexes — but they function as an integrated pair. Adequate niacin with depleted riboflavin still produces a crippled system, and vice versa. The orchestra cannot perform on half its string section.

Pantothenic Acid — The Gate's Key

Pantothenic acid — vitamin B5 — is the structural component of coenzyme A (CoA). Acetyl-CoA — the molecule that enters the Krebs cycle from pyruvate — cannot exist without CoA, and CoA cannot exist without pantothenic acid. The name derives from the

Greek for everywhere, which is precisely where it is found in food. Isolated deficiency is rare. But pantothenic acid is depleted by food processing, by alcohol, and by conditions of metabolic stress. And because its role is so central — without CoA, fats, carbohydrates, and proteins cannot all enter the energy production system — even modest insufficiency creates a broad metabolic bottleneck that does not announce itself with a specific diagnostic signature.

Pantothenic acid is also required for the synthesis of acetylcholine — the primary neurotransmitter of the parasympathetic nervous system, responsible for the rest-and-digest functions that chronic stress chronically suppresses. A person running on chronically elevated cortisol, eating a processed food diet, and relying on the parasympathetic nervous system to regulate digestion, heart rate, and anxiety is simultaneously depleting the vitamin that builds both the energy molecule and the calming neurotransmitter. The two deficits compound each other in ways that produce a clinical picture — fatigue, poor stress resilience, digestive dysfunction, anxiety — that generates diagnoses rather than upstream investigations.

Its essential partner: B5 works within the B-vitamin complex throughout the Krebs cycle. Thiamine, riboflavin, niacin, and B5 are all required for the full function of the pyruvate dehydrogenase complex and the Krebs cycle enzymes. They are not interchangeable soloists. They are a section, and the section must be complete.

Magnesium — The Activation Key

Magnesium deserves a book of its own — and has received several. Its role in the energy orchestra is singular but not singular enough. It functions at three distinct points in the energy production system: as a cofactor for glycolytic enzymes in Stage One, as a cofactor for Krebs cycle enzymes in Stage Two, and — most importantly — as the molecule that must bind to every ATP produced in Stage Three before that ATP can be used by anything in the body.

This last point is not trivial. ATP exists in the cell not as a free molecule but as a magnesium-ATP complex — MgATP. All the ATP-dependent processes in the body — every enzyme that requires ATP to function, every cellular pump that uses ATP to move ions, every kinase that uses ATP to phosphorylate a protein — they all require magnesium to unlock the ATP they depend on. Magnesium is not merely a nutrient that supports energy production. It is the key that activates every unit of energy the body makes.

The scale of magnesium's relevance to human health is staggering and almost entirely unappreciated in routine clinical practice. It is a cofactor for more than three hundred enzymes. It regulates calcium channels in muscle cells — magnesium insufficiency allows excess calcium influx, producing the muscle cramps, hypertension, and arterial spasm that are among the most common clinical presentations never investigated for their nutritional root. It governs NMDA receptor function in the brain — insufficient magnesium removes the protective block on these receptors, producing neuronal hyperexcitability that expresses itself as anxiety, insomnia, and migraine.

Serum magnesium — the test routinely ordered when magnesium is checked at all — measures the magnesium circulating in the blood, which represents less than one percent of total body magnesium. The body maintains serum magnesium at the expense of intracellular and bone stores, drawing down its reserves to keep the circulating level appearing normal for as long as possible. A serum magnesium within the laboratory reference range is therefore entirely compatible with significant intracellular magnesium deficiency. The appropriate test is red blood cell magnesium, which reflects intracellular status. It is almost never ordered.

Its essential partners: Magnesium depends on adequate vitamin D for its absorption — another nutrient dependency whose circularity has clinical consequences. Vitamin D supplementation without adequate magnesium is less effective because magnesium is required for the enzymatic conversion of vitamin D to its active form. Supplementing vitamin D in a magnesium-deficient patient may raise 25(OH)D levels modestly while leaving the clinical picture unchanged, because the active hormone cannot be produced. The two must be considered together.

Iron — The Structural Scaffolding

Iron is most familiar as the mineral at the center of hemoglobin — the protein that gives red blood cells their oxygen-carrying capacity. That role is real and important. But iron's role in the energy orchestra extends well beyond oxygen transport into the molecular architecture of the electron transport chain itself.

Iron-sulfur clusters — precisely engineered molecular structures containing iron and sulfur atoms — are the scaffolding through which electrons are passed between the complexes of the electron transport chain. Complex I contains eight iron-sulfur clusters. Complex II contains three. Complex III contains one. These clusters are not passive scaffolding. They are the electron-transfer chemistry. Without them, the electron transport chain cannot move electrons between its components.

Iron is also the metal at the center of the heme groups in cytochrome c — the protein that carries electrons from Complex III to Complex IV — and in the heme components of Complex IV itself. Iron deficiency does not merely produce anemia by reducing oxygen-carrying capacity. It reduces energy production at a more fundamental level by impairing the structural integrity of the electron transport chain, long before anemia develops and long before any routine blood test would identify a problem.

The subtlety here matters enormously for clinical practice. A patient with fatigue, a normal hemoglobin, and a ferritin of twenty micrograms per liter may be told their iron is fine. But ferritin — the storage form — may be normal in the early stages of iron depletion, while tissue iron — including the iron in mitochondrial enzyme complexes — is already insufficient. And ferritin, like magnesium and copper, is an acute-phase reactant that rises during inflammation, potentially masking underlying depletion. The complete picture requires transferrin saturation, serum iron, and TIBC interpreted in the context of inflammatory markers — a panel that requires a clinician who has been taught to look.

Its essential partner: Copper and iron have a relationship so intimate that they cannot be understood in isolation. The protein ceruloplasmin — which requires copper for its function — converts stored iron from the ferrous form in which it is stored to the ferric form in which it can be loaded onto transferrin for transport. Copper deficiency therefore produces iron deficiency anemia regardless of iron intake, because the iron cannot be mobilized. A patient treated for iron-deficiency anemia that does not respond to iron supplementation should be investigated for copper status. This is rarely done.

Copper — The Terminal Gate

Copper is the nutrient whose role in energy production has the greatest claim to being underappreciated in all of medicine, and whose deficit may be the most consequential single insufficiency driving the modern chronic disease burden. That claim requires justification, and the justification lies in the precise molecular role copper plays in Complex IV of the electron transport chain.

Cytochrome c oxidase — Complex IV — is the final complex in the electron transport chain. Its job is to accept electrons from cytochrome c and transfer them to molecular oxygen, reducing it to water. This is the reaction that collapses the electrochemical gradient and drives ATP synthase. Copper is not a cofactor for this enzyme in the conventional sense of a removable helper molecule. Two copper atoms — designated CuA and CuB — are structurally incorporated into the enzyme's active site. They are the chemistry that makes the electron transfer to oxygen physically possible.

Without copper, Complex IV cannot catalyze its reaction. The electron transport chain ends one complex too early. Electrons back up into Complex III, where electron leakage dramatically increases, producing a surge of superoxide free radicals — the most damaging class of reactive oxygen species the mitochondrion generates.

The consequences cascade through every high-energy-demanding tissue in the body simultaneously. The brain, which consumes approximately twenty percent of the body's energy despite comprising only two percent of its weight, is among the first to feel the deficit. Neurons begin to lose their myelin sheaths — the insulating layer that allows electrical signals to travel efficiently — because myelin maintenance is itself energy-intensive and because copper is independently required for the enzyme that builds myelin. The spinal cord deteriorates in a pattern indistinguishable from vitamin B12 deficiency — a clinical trap that has misled diagnosis in countless cases. The heart muscle, which never stops requiring ATP, weakens. The immune system, whose neutrophil count depends on copper-dependent bone marrow function, contracts.

Copper deficiency is considered rare. The data that would allow estimation of its true prevalence in subclinical form — RBC copper, superoxide dismutase activity — is almost never collected. What is collected — serum copper — is confounded by inflammation, which raises ceruloplasmin and therefore raises apparent serum copper regardless of true status. The mineral that sits at the final gate of the energy-producing process that every cell depends on is essentially unmeasured in standard medical practice.

Its essential partners: Copper and zinc compete for absorption through the same intestinal transporter, metallothionein. High-dose zinc supplementation — now extraordinarily common among health-conscious consumers, who take zinc for immune support, skin health, or testosterone optimization — reliably depletes copper over time. The person who has been taking fifty milligrams of zinc daily for two years while eating a diet moderate in liver and shellfish may have driven their copper status into functional insufficiency without any clinical investigation ever having been triggered. The copper-zinc balance, rather than either mineral in isolation, is the clinically relevant measure.

Zinc — The Structural Precision Instrument

Zinc appears in the energy orchestra in a supporting but non-negotiable role. It is a cofactor for glyceraldehyde-3-phosphate dehydrogenase, the enzyme that catalyzes one of the most energy-producing steps of glycolysis. It contributes to the structural integrity of Complex IV alongside copper. And it is the mineral partner in the superoxide dismutase enzyme — Cu/Zn-SOD — that neutralizes the superoxide radicals generated at Complexes I and III of the electron transport chain.

Zinc's broader significance to this chapter lies in its intimate antagonism with copper. Because zinc and copper share the same intestinal uptake mechanism, they exist in a biological tug of war. An adequate dietary copper-to-zinc ratio, estimated by many researchers at approximately one to eight, is essential for both minerals to be absorbed in functional amounts. The modern supplement market, by promoting high-dose zinc without an equivalent emphasis on copper, has created a population-level experiment in copper depletion that has no historical precedent and whose consequences are entirely unmeasured.

Its essential partner: Copper is zinc's essential partner in energy metabolism, and the ratio between them matters more than the absolute amount of either. The appropriate investigation is not zinc alone or copper alone but both, alongside the copper-zinc ratio.

Potassium — The Membrane Voltage

Potassium's contribution to the energy orchestra is foundational in a way that rarely receives acknowledgement. ATP synthase — the molecular turbine at the end of the electron transport chain that produces ATP from the proton gradient — depends on that gradient being maintained across the inner mitochondrial membrane. The gradient is electrochemical: it involves both a difference in hydrogen ion concentration and a difference in electrical charge across the membrane. Potassium is the primary determinant of that electrical charge differential in the cell.

When potassium is insufficient, the electrochemical conditions that drive ATP synthase are compromised. Energy production is impaired not by a missing enzyme cofactor but by the failure of the physical conditions that allow the chemistry to occur. Simultaneously, every nerve and muscle cell in the body — which use potassium gradients across their membranes to generate action potentials — becomes less able to function. The muscle weakness, cardiac arrhythmia, and profound fatigue of hypokalemia are not caused by failure of a specific enzyme. They are caused by the failure of the electrochemical physics of cellular function.

Its essential partner: Magnesium is required for the activity of the sodium-potassium ATPase pump — the enzyme that maintains potassium inside cells. Magnesium deficiency therefore produces intracellular potassium depletion even when dietary potassium is adequate, and potassium supplementation in a magnesium-deficient patient will be only partially effective because the pump that keeps potassium inside the cell cannot run properly without its magnesium cofactor.

Coenzyme Q10 — The Mobile Messenger

CoQ10 — ubiquinone — is the molecule that connects the first two complexes of the electron transport chain to the third. Without it, the electrons extracted from food by Complexes I and II have no way to reach Complex III and therefore cannot continue their journey toward ATP production. CoQ10 is the courier between the loading docks and the factory floor.

It also functions in its reduced form — ubiquinol — as a fat-soluble antioxidant, neutralizing lipid peroxyl radicals in the inner mitochondrial membrane. It is therefore simultaneously essential for energy production and essential for protecting the membrane in which the energy-producing machinery is embedded. Deplete

CoQ10 and the factory produces less product while the factory walls degrade faster.

CoQ10 is not obtained primarily from diet — most is synthesized by the body. But that synthesis depends on a pathway — the mevalonate pathway — that statins, the most widely prescribed class of drugs in the world, directly block. Statin therapy reduces CoQ10 synthesis in proportion to its LDL-reducing effect. The myopathy — muscle pain and weakness — experienced by five to twenty percent of statin users is biochemically consistent with CoQ10 depletion in skeletal muscle. The cardiac implications are more concerning: a drug prescribed to protect the heart reduces the production of the electron carrier that cardiac muscle, the most mitochondria-dense tissue in the body, depends on most. This interaction has been documented repeatedly in the scientific literature and is addressed almost never in the clinical conversation between prescribing physician and patient.

Its essential partners: CoQ10 synthesis requires the mevalonate pathway and therefore depends on adequate B vitamins and magnesium throughout the pathway. Selenium is required for the recycling of ubiquinol back to ubiquinone. The antioxidant function of CoQ10 is integrated with vitamin E and vitamin C — each regenerating the others in a network that requires all of them to function.

Carnitine — The Fat Transporter

Of the approximately forty kilograms of ATP the human body produces daily, a substantial proportion is derived not from carbohydrate but from fat. Beta-oxidation — the breakdown of fatty acids for energy — is a major fuel pathway, particularly for heart muscle and skeletal muscle during sustained activity. Fatty acids cannot enter the mitochondria on their own. They must be attached to carnitine, which escorts them across the inner mitochondrial membrane. Without carnitine, fatty acid fuel cannot reach the furnace.

Carnitine is synthesized in the body from two amino acids — lysine and methionine — but the synthesis requires three additional nutrients: vitamin C, iron, and vitamin B6. This multi-nutrient dependency of carnitine synthesis is one of the clearest illustrations of the interconnected nature of the energy orchestra: a single missing musician in the carnitine synthesis pathway renders the entire fat fuel delivery system less efficient, regardless of the adequacy of every other component.

Carnitine deficiency produces a clinical picture dominated by profound muscle weakness and cardiac muscle dysfunction — reflecting the dependence of these high-fat-oxidizing tissues on carnitine-mediated fatty acid delivery. The picture is consistent with a condition medicine has no nutritional framework for identifying because it does not test for carnitine status, does not assess the B6, vitamin C, and iron status required for its synthesis, and does not connect the dots between them.

Its essential partners: The carnitine synthesis chain — lysine + methionine + vitamin C + iron + vitamin B6 — is one of the best demonstrations in this book of how nutritional deficiencies multiply. Each link in this chain is a musician. The fat transport system performs at the level of its weakest member.

PQQ — The Mitochondrial Architect

Pyrroloquinoline quinone — PQQ — is the least well known nutrient in this chapter and among the most significant for the future of energy medicine. It is found in trace amounts in breast milk, fermented foods, and certain vegetables, and it performs a function no other nutritional compound is known to perform: it stimulates mitochondrial biogenesis — the creation of entirely new mitochondria.

Every other nutrient in this chapter supports the function of existing mitochondria. PQQ builds new ones. A person whose mitochondrial population has been depleted by years of nutritional insufficiency, chronic illness, or aging does not simply need better-functioning mitochondria. They need more of them. PQQ activates the transcription factors — PGC-1α and NRF-1 and NRF-2 — that govern the expression of genes required to build new mitochondrial membranes, new electron transport chain complexes, and new mitochondrial DNA.

PQQ is also a catalytic antioxidant of extraordinary potency — a molecule that can perform thousands of oxidation-reduction cycles before it is degraded, compared to vitamin C which performs one and must be regenerated. Inside the cell, it protects the very mitochondria it is also helping to build.

Clinical research on PQQ is in its early stages relative to the more established members of this cluster. But the foundational science is clear, the safety record is good, and the logic of its role — in a world where mitochondrial depletion is a plausible consequence of the modern lifestyle — is compelling. It belongs in this chapter because an orchestra cannot perform its best with diminished numbers, and PQQ is currently the only identified nutritional conductor capable of calling new musicians to the stage.

Its essential partners: PQQ's mitochondrial biogenesis function works in concert with CoQ10 — new mitochondria require CoQ10 to function from the moment they are assembled. The two nutrients together address both the quality and the quantity of mitochondrial energy production capacity.

VI. Why the Orchestra Is Playing Short-Staffed

The energy orchestra described above has operated without significant attrition for most of human history. The diets of pre-industrial populations — varied, whole-food, mineral-rich, fermented, seasonal, and low in refined carbohydrates — supplied the full complement of energy nutrients in the forms and ratios the body evolved to utilize. The mitochondria of a traditional diet were playing a full ensemble.

Modern life has systematically removed musicians from the stage through five overlapping mechanisms, none of which is individually catastrophic but whose cumulative effect — across an entire population, across a lifetime — represents a genuine nutritional crisis that the medical system is not structured to see.

Soil and Food Depletion

Intensive agricultural practices over the past century have progressively depleted the mineral content of arable soils. Studies comparing the nutrient density of fruits and vegetables grown in the same regions in the 1940s versus the 1990s found declines of twenty to eighty percent for minerals including iron, copper, magnesium, and zinc. A person eating the same diet as their grandparents — same foods, same quantities — is receiving meaningfully less of every mineral in this chapter. The food has not changed in appearance. The nutritional content has.

Food Processing

Refining removes the outer layers of grains where the greatest concentrations of B vitamins, minerals, and CoQ10 precursors reside. The milling process that produces white flour removes approximately seventy-seven percent of the thiamine, eighty percent of the riboflavin, eighty-one percent of the niacin, and sixty percent of the magnesium from the original grain. Fortification replaces a fraction of what is lost, selectively. The net effect is that populations eating primarily processed food are running the energy orchestra on a systematically stripped-down score.

The Zinc Supplement Problem

The widespread use of high-dose zinc supplements — for immune support, for skin health, for testosterone, for viral illness — has created a population-level copper depletion experiment with no historical precedent. Doses above 40mg/day consumed over months reliably reduce copper absorption. Doses that are commonly available over the counter, commonly recommended online, and commonly taken by health-conscious individuals. The copper that sits at the terminal gate of the electron transport chain is being displaced by an unmanaged supplement practice that medicine has not recognized as a public health concern.

Medications That Deplete

Several of the most commonly prescribed medications in the developed world have documented nutrient-depleting effects directly relevant to this chapter. Beta-blockers reduce CoQ10 through the mevalonate pathway. Proton pump inhibitors impair the absorption of magnesium, iron, zinc, and thiamine. Loop diuretics deplete thiamine, magnesium, and potassium. Statins reduce CoQ10. Metformin depletes B12, which indirectly affects the methylation of mitochondrial DNA. These are not theoretical interactions. They are documented, published, and clinically ignored.

Chronic Stress

Chronic psychological and physiological stress activates the hypothalamic-pituitary-adrenal axis and the sympathetic nervous system, both of which accelerate the metabolic demand for energy nutrients. Thiamine demand rises with carbohydrate metabolism rate, which chronic stress drives upward. Magnesium is excreted in the urine in proportion to cortisol levels — chronic stress is a chronic magnesium drain. Vitamin C is consumed by the adrenal glands in the synthesis of cortisol and adrenaline. The more a person needs their energy metabolism to support them under stress, the faster they deplete the nutrients that run it.

> *The perfect modern lifestyle for depleting the energy orchestra looks like this: a processed-food diet, high in refined carbohydrates, low in organ meats and shellfish. Regular zinc supplementation without copper. A prescription for a proton pump inhibitor for occasional reflux. A statin for borderline cholesterol. A demanding job and insufficient sleep. This is not an unusual life. It is an ordinary one. And it produces, over years, the kind of fatigue that fills the waiting rooms of clinicians who have no nutritional framework for understanding it.*

VII. The Web of Dependencies

The nutrients in this chapter are not independent interventions that happen to share a metabolic address. They are a network, and the network has a topology. Understanding the topology is what separates the upstream thinker from the downstream treater.

Thiamine cannot be activated without magnesium. Magnesium cannot be properly absorbed without vitamin D. Vitamin D cannot be converted to its active form without magnesium — a circular dependency that means deficiency in either tends to perpetuate the other. Iron cannot be mobilized from storage without copper-dependent ceruloplasmin. Copper absorption is suppressed by excess zinc. Zinc absorption is impaired by gut dysbiosis. Carnitine cannot be synthesized without vitamin C, iron, and B6 — each of which has its own dependency network. CoQ10 production requires the mevalonate pathway that statins block. PQQ stimulates the mitochondrial biogenesis that requires CoQ10 to populate the new mitochondria being built.

This is not a list of interactions to be memorized. It is an argument for a different way of thinking about nutritional sufficiency. A clinician who tests a single marker and finds it within the reference range has not established nutritional adequacy. They have established that one musician, checked in isolation, passed the audition. The concert still requires the full ensemble.

The drug-nutrient interactions that deplete this cluster deserve particular emphasis because they represent an iatrogenic layer of energy insufficiency added on top of dietary insufficiency. A patient taking a proton pump inhibitor for gastro-esophageal reflux is impairing the absorption of magnesium, thiamine, iron, and zinc simultaneously. A patient taking a statin for elevated LDL is blocking the synthesis of CoQ10 in the very cardiac muscle the statin is prescribed to protect. A patient taking a loop diuretic for hypertension is excreting thiamine, magnesium, and potassium in the urine. The fatigue these patients experience is documented, attributed to their underlying conditions, and treated with reassurance. The nutritional mechanism is present, identifiable, and unaddressed.

VIII. Questions Worth Asking

This chapter is not a treatment protocol. The information it contains is presented to inform, not to prescribe, and nothing here should substitute for the individualized assessment of a qualified healthcare professional. What it offers, instead, are the questions that the conventional medical encounter does not currently ask — and that the evidence suggests are worth raising.

For a person experiencing unexplained fatigue — the kind that persists despite adequate sleep, that does not respond to thyroid management, that blood work consistently fails to explain — the following represent a starting point for a different kind of conversation. Not a supplement protocol. A testing conversation.

Red blood cell magnesium, rather than serum magnesium, provides a clinically meaningful picture of intracellular magnesium status. Serum magnesium within the normal range does not exclude intracellular deficiency. Red blood cell copper and serum ceruloplasmin together provide a more complete picture of copper status than serum copper alone, which is confounded by inflammation. Ferritin interpreted alongside transferrin saturation, serum iron, and C-reactive protein gives a more complete picture of iron status than ferritin in isolation. Whole blood thiamine or transketolase activity reflects functional thiamine status better than serum thiamine. And in a patient taking a statin, beta-blocker, proton pump inhibitor, or loop diuretic, a conversation about the nutrient-depleting effects of these medications — and whether monitoring or support is indicated — is a conversation that the evidence supports and the clinical encounter rarely includes.

The nutrients discussed in this chapter are not presented as treatments for any medical condition. They are presented as components of normal physiological function whose insufficiency may contribute to the symptoms described, and whose assessment may inform conversations with a qualified healthcare professional. The author of this book is not a clinician and does not offer clinical advice. All testing and any decisions based on it should be undertaken with appropriate professional guidance.

IX. Margaret's Orchestra, Heard Properly

Margaret's fatigue, reconsidered through the lens of this chapter, stops being a mystery and becomes a diagnosis written in nutritional shorthand.

Her proton pump inhibitor — prescribed three years ago for reflux and continued indefinitely — has been silently reducing her absorption of magnesium, thiamine, iron, and zinc throughout. Her beta-blocker — prescribed for hypertension that may itself reflect magnesium insufficiency — has been suppressing her CoQ10 synthesis throughout the same period, impairing the mitochondrial electron transport on which her cardiac muscle depends. Her high-carbohydrate diet — low in organ meats, low in shellfish, low in the dense mineral and B-vitamin sources her energy orchestra requires — has been under-supplying thiamine relative to the carbohydrate load it is being asked to metabolize. Her decade of chronic stress has been driving magnesium out through the kidneys at an accelerated rate and consuming vitamin C in the adrenal glands that are synthesizing the cortisol required to manage it.

The orchestra has been playing short-staffed for years. The musicians who remain have been compensating — the body is extraordinarily good at compensation, at maintaining apparent function while true capacity quietly erodes — until the compensation is no longer sufficient and the fatigue becomes the only signal loud enough to hear.

Nobody told Margaret that the combination of her diet, her medications, and her decade of stress represented a systematic depletion of the nutrients that power her cells. Nobody measured the nutrients in question. Nobody connected the prescription to the depletion to the symptom. The tools existed. The knowledge existed. The question was never asked.

What Margaret deserved was not a different answer to the question her physicians asked. She deserved a physician who had been trained to ask a different question: not what is wrong, but what is missing. Not which diagnosis applies, but what the energy orchestra is playing on, and what it is missing, and whether those missing elements might explain what three years of blood work have failed to find.

For the Clinically Curious

The Pyruvate Dehydrogenase Complex — Molecular Architecture

The pyruvate dehydrogenase complex (PDC) is a multi-enzyme assembly of three catalytic components (E1, E2, E3) and two regulatory proteins. E1 (pyruvate decarboxylase) requires thiamine pyrophosphate (TPP) at its active site and cannot function in its absence. E2 (dihydrolipoyl transacetylase) requires lipoic acid — a cofactor that must be regenerated after each catalytic cycle, a process requiring NADH (niacin-derived) and FAD (riboflavin-derived). E3 (dihydrolipoyl dehydrogenase) requires FAD and NAD+. The complete PDC therefore requires thiamine, lipoic acid, riboflavin, and niacin functioning together — any single insufficiency produces PDC dysfunction. This is the molecular basis for the clinical observation that the B vitamins act as a group rather than as independent variables.

Iron-Sulfur Clusters — The Electron Transfer Architecture

Iron-sulfur (Fe-S) clusters are molecular modules of iron and sulfur atoms that adopt different oxidation states to transfer electrons through the electron transport chain. Complex I contains eight Fe-S clusters (one 2Fe-2S and seven 4Fe-4S); Complex II contains three Fe-S clusters; Complex III contains one Rieske Fe-S cluster. Their assembly requires dedicated chaperone proteins and a sulfur source — dietary sulfur from methionine, cysteine, and the transsulfuration pathway. Iron deficiency impairs Fe-S cluster assembly and therefore ETC function independently of anemia, typically at tissue ferritin levels that remain within laboratory reference ranges.

Cytochrome c Oxidase — The Copper Chemistry

CuA in Complex IV is a binuclear copper center that receives electrons from cytochrome c. CuB, paired with a heme iron (heme a3), forms the binuclear center at which molecular oxygen is reduced to water. The CuB-heme a3 center binds O_2 and orchestrates a four-electron reduction that prevents the release of partially reduced oxygen species (superoxide, hydrogen peroxide, hydroxyl radical). Copper insufficiency at Complex IV therefore produces two simultaneous pathological consequences: reduced ATP production as electron flow stalls, and increased reactive oxygen species generation as electrons leak from earlier complexes whose output cannot be accepted downstream.

MgATP — Why Magnesium Is the Activation Key

Virtually all enzymatic reactions that utilize ATP actually utilize MgATP — the chelate formed between magnesium and the triphosphate moiety of ATP. The magnesium ion stabilizes the negative charges on the phosphate groups and positions the terminal phosphate for nucleophilic attack by the enzyme's substrate. Kinases, ATPases, synthetases, and ligases all require MgATP rather than free ATP. In the context of intracellular magnesium depletion, the body may be producing adequate ATP while that ATP is functionally unavailable — energy produced but not deployed. This is consistent with the clinical presentation of magnesium insufficiency, in which fatigue and reduced exercise capacity occur against a background of apparently normal cellular energy substrate availability.

CoQ10 Depletion by Statins — The Pharmacological Mechanism

Statins inhibit HMG-CoA reductase, the rate-limiting enzyme of the mevalonate pathway. The mevalonate pathway produces not only cholesterol but also the isoprenoid precursors (farnesyl pyrophosphate and geranylgeranyl pyrophosphate) required for CoQ10 side-chain synthesis. Statin-induced CoQ10 depletion is proportional to the degree of HMG-CoA reductase inhibition. Skeletal muscle mitochondrial CoQ10 concentrations have been documented to decline by forty to fifty percent with statin therapy in some studies. The clinical threshold at which this reduction produces symptomatic myopathy varies with baseline CoQ10 status, mitochondrial reserve capacity, and muscle metabolic demand. Routine monitoring of CoQ10 status in statin-treated patients is not currently a clinical standard despite the documented pharmacological mechanism.

Functional Testing — What to Measure and Why

Standard metabolic panels do not assess any of the twelve nutrients in this cluster in a clinically meaningful way. The following functional tests provide superior clinical information: (1) RBC magnesium (intracellular status, not confounded by homeostatic maintenance of serum levels); (2) Whole blood thiamine or erythrocyte transketolase activity (functional assessment, not serum thiamine which is unreliable); (3) RBC copper plus serum ceruloplasmin plus Cu/Zn-SOD activity (the triad provides functional copper status uncoupled from acute-phase elevation of ceruloplasmin); (4) Serum ferritin + transferrin saturation + serum iron + TIBC + CRP (the full iron panel, interpreted together, in inflammatory context); (5) Serum or plasma CoQ10 (particularly indicated in statin-treated patients); (6) Plasma carnitine (total and free); (7) Serum B vitamins where indicated by clinical picture. The absence of these tests from routine panels is not evidence that they are unnecessary — it is evidence that they are not yet standard, which is a different claim.

---

* * *

The energy orchestra plays in every cell of every person alive. It plays continuously, without rest, without interruption, from the first moment of fetal life to the last beat of the heart. It requires twelve musicians to play their parts in precise coordination, each dependent on the others, each irreplaceable in its own section of the score.

Modern life has been quietly removing musicians from the stage. Not dramatically — no single depletion is sufficient to collapse the orchestra immediately. But gradually, over years, as dietary quality declines, as medications accumulate, as stress mounts and gut function deteriorates and supplements are taken without balance — the ensemble shrinks. The music that remains is recognizable as energy. But it is not the full piece. And the fatigue that results — the unexplained, persistent, blood-work-normal fatigue of millions of patients like Margaret — is the sound of a performance being given by an orchestra that is no longer complete.

The musicians are identifiable. Their absence is measurable. And the question of whether they are present in adequate numbers is one that the right tests, asked of the right clinician, can begin to answer.

The next chapter asks a prior question: before any of these musicians can perform, the concert hall itself must be functional. The gut — the master gateway through which every nutrient in this book must pass — is where every orchestra begins.

Cluster 2

The Master Gateway

How the Gut Determines Whether Every Other Musician in the Orchestra Gets to Perform

"All disease begins in the gut."

— Hippocrates, c. 400 BCE — a statement whose molecular basis is only now being understood

---

I. The Door Everything Must Pass Through

Margaret had been taking her medications faithfully for three years. The thyroid medication. The blood pressure tablets. The magnesium supplement her most recent physician had suggested after finally ordering an RBC magnesium. She had adjusted her diet, reduced processed foods, added leafy greens. By every measure available to her, she was doing the right things. And yet the fatigue persisted, the anxiety remained, and her follow-up bloods showed nutrient levels stubbornly unchanged.

Nobody had asked about her gut. Nobody had considered that between the nutrients she was consuming and the cells that needed them stood a gatekeeper that the medical system had spent a century ignoring: the intestinal lining — one cell thick, spanning a surface area the size of a singles tennis court if unfolded, responsible for determining which molecules from the outside world are invited into the body and which are not.

The gut is not a passive tube. It is the most sophisticated molecular selection system in biology. And in Margaret — after four courses of antibiotics, three years on a proton pump inhibitor, a decade of chronic stress, and a processed-food diet — that system was not performing its selection function properly. The nutrients she was consuming were passing through an impaired gateway. Some were not making it through at all.

This chapter comes early in the book because it must. Before any of the other clusters can be fully understood, the reader needs to understand the gateway through which every musician in the orchestra must pass before they can take their place on stage. Heal the gateway, and every subsequent intervention becomes more effective. Ignore it, and every subsequent intervention works at a fraction of its potential.

II. Meet the Cast

Ten musicians make up the gut gateway orchestra described in this chapter. Each plays a distinct role in maintaining the integrity, selectivity, and function of the gut as the master portal of nutritional entry.

- **Glutamine** — The primary fuel for enterocytes — the cells lining the gut wall. The intestinal lining renews itself every three to five days, making it one of the most rapidly dividing tissues in the body and one of the most glutamine-hungry.
- **Zinc** — The mineral that maintains the tight junctions — the molecular seals between adjacent gut lining cells — that determine what passes through and what does not.
- **Vitamin D** — The immune regulator within the gut's vast mucosal immune system, calibrating the balance between tolerance of food and beneficial bacteria and defense against pathogens.
- **Vitamin A** — The guardian of the mucosal barrier, governing the differentiation of the epithelial cells that form the gut lining and the mucus-producing goblet cells above them.
- **Butyrate** — The short-chain fatty acid produced by bacterial fermentation of dietary fiber that serves as the primary fuel for colonocytes in the large intestine and the primary anti-inflammatory signal keeping the colonic immune system calm.
- **Threonine** — The amino acid most concentrated in intestinal mucin — the protective mucus layer that coats the gut wall. Without adequate threonine, the mucus layer thins, and the distance between the gut contents and the epithelial cells below it decreases.
- **Glycine** — Structural component of the collagen in the gut's basement membrane, cofactor in gut lining repair, and anti-inflammatory molecule that suppresses NF-κB activation in intestinal immune cells.

- **Omega-3 fatty acids** — Anti-inflammatory modulators of the gut's prostaglandin balance, reducing the production of pro-inflammatory eicosanoids that drive intestinal permeability and mucosal damage.
- **Vitamin C** — Collagen synthesis support for the gut's structural matrix, antioxidant protection for intestinal epithelial cells, and cofactor for the enzymes that maintain gut barrier integrity.
- **Phosphatidylcholine** — The dominant phospholipid of the intestinal mucus layer, particularly in the colon. Depletion — documented in inflammatory bowel disease — reduces the hydrophobic barrier that prevents bacteria from reaching the epithelium.

These ten musicians do not operate independently. Together they maintain what medicine is only beginning to appreciate as one of the most consequential biological structures in human health: a gut wall that is simultaneously permeable enough to absorb nutrients and selective enough to exclude what should not enter the bloodstream.

III. The Concert Hall: How the Gut Works

The intestinal wall is constructed in layers. At the outermost surface — the layer in contact with the gut contents — sits the mucus layer, a thick gel of glycoproteins secreted by goblet cells embedded throughout the epithelium. This layer is the gut's first line of defense: a physical barrier that keeps bacteria at a safe distance from the epithelial cells below, and a chemical environment that traps and neutralizes potential pathogens while allowing nutrients to pass through.

Beneath the mucus layer lies the single layer of epithelial cells — enterocytes — that forms the actual wall of the intestine. These cells are joined to each other by tight junctions: protein complexes that seal the spaces between adjacent cells, creating a continuous barrier through which only selectively permitted molecules can pass. The tight junctions are not fixed structures. They open and close in response to signals from the gut contents, the immune system, the microbiome, and the nutritional status of the enterocytes themselves.

Below the epithelium lies the lamina propria — a layer rich in immune cells, including the vast mucosal immune system that makes the gut the largest immune organ in the body. Approximately seventy percent of the body's immune tissue lines the gut. This concentration reflects the scale of the immunological challenge: every day, the gut must distinguish between the trillions of commensal bacteria that belong there, the harmless food proteins that must be tolerated, and the pathogens and toxins that must be repelled. The calibration of this distinction is one of the most sophisticated biological processes in human physiology. And it is directly dependent on the nutritional status of the gut wall.

What Happens When the Gateway Fails

When the tight junctions between enterocytes loosen — a condition described as increased intestinal permeability, and colloquially as leaky gut — the selective barrier becomes non-selective. Bacterial fragments, partially digested food proteins, and microbial toxins including lipopolysaccharide (LPS) — a component of bacterial cell walls that is a potent immune activator — translocate from the gut lumen into the lamina propria and from there into the systemic circulation.

The immune system encounters LPS and mounts an inflammatory response. In the short term, this is appropriate and necessary — LPS signals infection. But when LPS translocation becomes chronic — when increased permeability allows a continuous low-level leak of bacterial fragments into the bloodstream — the immune system sustains a chronic low-grade inflammatory state. This state has been mechanistically linked to depression, Alzheimer's disease, cardiovascular disease, metabolic syndrome, autoimmune conditions, and fatigue syndromes. It is called endotoxemia, and it is one of the most important and least discussed mechanisms through which gut dysfunction produces systemic disease.

> *A gut wall that is one cell thick, spanning a surface area the size of a singles tennis court, maintained by nutrients that most people never hear about and no physician routinely measures — this is the gateway between the outside world and every cell in the human body. Its integrity is not a gastroenterological concern.*

> *It is the central architectural requirement of human health.*

IV. The Musicians, One by One

Glutamine — The Enterocyte's Primary Fuel

The cells lining the small intestine — enterocytes — renew themselves completely every three to five days, making the gut lining one of the most rapidly dividing tissues in the body. This extraordinary rate of cellular renewal requires an extraordinary supply of energy substrate, and the preferred fuel of enterocytes is not glucose, as one might expect, but glutamine — a conditionally essential amino acid that becomes the primary energy source for intestinal cells under conditions of normal function and especially under conditions of stress, illness, or injury.

When glutamine supply is insufficient — during critical illness, prolonged fasting, intensive exercise, or dietary inadequacy — enterocyte renewal slows, the gut lining thins, and the tight junctions between cells begin to loosen. The gateway becomes less selective. Studies in surgical and critical care patients have documented that glutamine supplementation reduces intestinal permeability, reduces bacterial translocation, reduces septic complications, and improves clinical outcomes. The gut lining is not resilient in the absence of its primary fuel.

Its essential partners: Glutamine requires adequate B6 for its metabolism and adequate zinc for the tight junction proteins it helps maintain. Vitamin D regulates the expression of genes involved in gut barrier function, including those governing the tight junction proteins that glutamine supports structurally. The trio of glutamine, zinc, and vitamin D forms the core of gut barrier nutritional support.

Zinc — The Tight Junction Keeper

Tight junctions are protein complexes — primarily occludin, claudins, and zonula occludens proteins — that bridge the space between adjacent enterocytes and determine the paracellular permeability of the gut wall. Zinc is required for the structural integrity and assembly of these complexes. Zinc deficiency loosens tight junctions and increases gut permeability; zinc repletion tightens them. The mechanism is direct and documented, and it means that every person with zinc insufficiency — which the widespread use of high-dose zinc supplements without copper may paradoxically be creating in some and correcting in others — has a gut lining that is less selective than it should be.

Zinc also regulates gut immune function as a cofactor for thymulin, the thymic hormone required for T-cell development, and for multiple enzymes in the mucosal immune system. A zinc-deficient gut is both more permeable and less immunologically competent — a combination that creates exactly the dysregulated immune environment from which autoimmune conditions emerge.

Its essential partners: Zinc and copper compete for the same intestinal transporter, metallothionein. Excess zinc suppresses copper absorption, and copper is required for the lysyl oxidase enzyme that maintains collagen integrity in the gut's basement membrane. The balance between zinc and copper matters in the gut as much as anywhere in the body.

Vitamin D — The Mucosal Immune Calibrator

Vitamin D receptors are expressed throughout the gastrointestinal tract — in enterocytes, in goblet cells, and in the immune cells of the lamina propria. The active form of vitamin D, 1,25-dihydroxyvitamin D3, regulates the expression of genes involved in gut barrier function including the tight junction proteins that determine permeability, and the defensins — antimicrobial peptides that form the gut's chemical defense layer above the epithelium.

Vitamin D deficiency is associated with increased intestinal permeability, reduced antimicrobial peptide production, altered microbiome composition, and increased susceptibility to inflammatory bowel disease. Vitamin D supplementation has been shown to reduce markers of intestinal permeability and improve symptoms in inflammatory bowel disease in multiple clinical trials. The gut is not a secondary site of vitamin D action. It is one of its primary targets.

Its essential partners: Vitamin D requires magnesium for its conversion to the active form in both the liver and kidney. The gut is also where vitamin D — a fat-soluble vitamin — must be absorbed, requiring adequate bile acids (themselves dependent on liver function and microbiome health) and dietary fat. A person with gut dysfunction may be unable to absorb the vitamin D that would help repair that dysfunction — a circular problem requiring both direct gut support and vitamin D repletion simultaneously.

Vitamin A — The Barrier Architect

Vitamin A — in its retinol and retinoic acid forms — is the master regulator of epithelial differentiation throughout the body. In the gut, retinoic acid governs the differentiation of goblet cells — the mucus-producing cells whose secretions form the protective layer above the epithelium — and regulates the expression of mucin genes. Without adequate vitamin A, goblet cell numbers decline, mucin production falls, and the mucus layer thins. The distance between gut bacteria and the epithelial cells below decreases. The structural first line of defense weakens.

Vitamin A also plays a critical role in mucosal immune regulation, driving the development of regulatory T cells and IgA-producing plasma cells in the gut-associated lymphoid tissue. Secretory IgA — the antibody that coats the mucosal surface and neutralizes pathogens before they reach the epithelium — depends on vitamin A for its production. A vitamin A-deficient gut is a gut with thin mucus, reduced IgA, and impaired regulatory immunity — the precise combination that characterizes inflammatory bowel disease and leaky gut.

Its essential partners: Vitamin A and vitamin D work together at nuclear receptors throughout the gut wall. The retinoid X receptor

(RXR) partners with the vitamin D receptor (VDR) to form heterodimers that regulate gene expression — meaning that adequate vitamin A is required for full vitamin D receptor function and vice versa. The fat-soluble vitamins are not independent variables. In the gut as elsewhere, they are an integrated system.

Butyrate — The Colonocyte's Lifeblood

Butyrate is a short-chain fatty acid produced by the bacterial fermentation of dietary fiber in the large intestine. It is the primary fuel for colonocytes — the cells lining the colon — providing approximately seventy percent of their energy requirements. But butyrate is far more than an energy source. It is a signaling molecule with profound effects on gene expression, immune regulation, and gut barrier integrity.

Butyrate inhibits histone deacetylases — enzymes that silence gene expression — and thereby promotes the expression of genes involved in cell differentiation, apoptosis of damaged cells, and anti-inflammatory signaling. It suppresses NF-κB, the master inflammatory transcription factor, reducing the production of pro-inflammatory cytokines in colonic immune cells. It promotes the development of regulatory T cells in the colonic lamina propria. And it directly tightens tight junctions, improving the physical barrier function of the colonic epithelium.

A colon without adequate butyrate production — the consequence of a fiber-depleted diet or a dysbiotic microbiome lacking butyrate-producing bacteria — is a colon running on emergency power. Its cells become more susceptible to DNA damage, its immune regulation shifts toward inflammation, and its barrier function degrades. The conditions for colorectal cancer, inflammatory bowel disease, and systemic endotoxemia are created by the absence of a molecule that a diverse, fiber-fed microbiome would produce automatically.

Its essential partners: Butyrate production requires both dietary fiber — the substrate for fermentation — and the specific gut bacteria (primarily Firmicutes species including Faecalibacterium prausnitzii and Roseburia intestinalis) that perform the fermentation. The microbiome chapter covers these relationships in depth. Butyrate also requires adequate vitamin D to upregulate the butyrate transporter in colonocytes, another example of the nutrient interdependency that characterizes every system in this book.

Threonine — The Mucus Layer's Foundation

Threonine is the most concentrated amino acid in intestinal mucin — the gel-forming glycoprotein that constitutes the protective mucus layer coating the gut wall. Mucin molecules are composed of protein backbones densely decorated with carbohydrate side chains, and the protein backbone is particularly rich in threonine, serine, and proline residues to which these chains attach. Approximately forty percent of the amino acids in mucin are threonine.

When dietary threonine is insufficient — as it frequently is in low-protein diets, in the elderly, in plant-based eaters who do not optimize their amino acid intake, and in anyone under significant metabolic stress — mucin synthesis is compromised before virtually any other protein synthesis in the body, because the gut lining cannot run on stored reserves. The mucus layer thins. The distance between the gut bacteria and the epithelial cells below decreases. The vulnerability to bacterial invasion and inflammatory activation increases.

This mechanism is almost never discussed clinically. Threonine is not on any standard blood panel. Its role in gut barrier integrity is documented in the research literature and absent from clinical practice. A person with recurrent gastrointestinal inflammation whose threonine intake has never been assessed represents the gap between what the science knows and what the clinical encounter addresses.

Its essential partner: Threonine works alongside glycine — which provides structural support for the collagen in the gut's basement membrane below the epithelium — and alongside glutamine, which fuels the enterocytes themselves. The gut lining requires adequate threonine for its mucus above, adequate collagen (glycine + proline + vitamin C + copper) for its basement membrane below, and adequate glutamine for the cells in between.

Glycine — The Anti-Inflammatory Structural Protein

Glycine is the most abundant amino acid in collagen, making up approximately thirty percent of collagen's total amino acid content. The gut wall rests on a collagen-rich basement membrane that provides structural support for the epithelium above it. When collagen synthesis is inadequate — due to insufficient glycine, or insufficient vitamin C, copper, or proline that collagen also requires — the basement membrane weakens, the structural support for the epithelial layer diminishes, and the gut wall becomes more fragile.

Beyond its structural role, glycine functions as an inhibitory neurotransmitter at glycine receptors in the enteric nervous system, modulating gut motility and the pain signaling that produces the visceral hypersensitivity characteristic of irritable bowel syndrome. And in the immune cells of the gut lamina propria, glycine directly inhibits NF-κB activation and reduces the production of inflammatory cytokines — making it one of the most potent anti-inflammatory amino acids in the gut immune system. Clinical studies have documented glycine's ability to reduce mucosal inflammation in models of colitis, and its anti-inflammatory properties are being explored in inflammatory bowel disease.

Its essential partners: Glycine is also a component of glutathione — alongside glutamate and cysteine — making it essential not only for gut structural integrity and immune regulation but for the antioxidant defense that protects the gut lining from oxidative damage. A glycine-depleted gut is simultaneously structurally weaker, more inflammatory, and less antioxidant-defended.

Omega-3 Fatty Acids — The Anti-Inflammatory Signal

The prostaglandin balance in the gut wall determines whether the mucosal immune response tends toward inflammation or resolution. Arachidonic acid — an omega-6 fatty acid — is the precursor to pro-inflammatory prostaglandin E2 and other eicosanoids that increase gut permeability and amplify immune activation. EPA — eicosapentaenoic acid, an omega-3 fatty acid — competes with arachidonic acid for the same enzymes, producing instead prostaglandin E3 and the anti-inflammatory resolvins and protectins that resolve rather than amplify inflammation.

The modern dietary omega-3 to omega-6 ratio of approximately 1:15 to 1:20 — compared to an ancestral ratio estimated at approximately 1:4 — systematically biases the gut's prostaglandin balance toward the inflammatory pathway. The gut wall of a person eating a modern Western diet is producing more pro-inflammatory eicosanoids and fewer resolving molecules than the gut wall evolved to receive. The result is a chronic low-grade inflammatory state in the gut mucosa that is not the dramatic inflammation of Crohn's disease but is nonetheless impairing barrier function, altering immune calibration, and contributing to the systemic endotoxemia that underlies so many chronic conditions.

Its essential partners: Omega-3 fatty acids require adequate vitamin E to prevent their oxidation — EPA and DHA are highly polyunsaturated and particularly vulnerable to lipid peroxidation. They also require vitamin D, which upregulates the resolvin synthesis pathway. And they depend on a healthy gut microbiome for their conversion to the most active anti-inflammatory mediators — resolvins and protectins — demonstrating once again that gut health and nutritional health are mutually dependent.

Vitamin C — The Gut's Structural Maintenance

Vitamin C is the cofactor for prolyl hydroxylase and lysyl hydroxylase — the enzymes that hydroxylate proline and lysine residues in collagen chains, a modification required for collagen to fold into its characteristic triple helix and for collagen fibers to cross-link into the structural matrix of the gut wall. Without vitamin C, collagen synthesis is impaired throughout the body — including in the gut's basement membrane and in the connective tissue of the lamina propria.

Vitamin C also functions as an antioxidant in the intestinal epithelium, protecting enterocytes from the oxidative stress generated by the constant processing of the gut's contents. And it is required for the absorption of non-heme iron in the small intestine — a role that makes it the single most important co-nutrient for iron bioavailability from plant sources, and that means that vitamin C insufficiency contributes to iron deficiency even when dietary iron intake is adequate.

Its essential partners: Vitamin C regenerates vitamin E after it has neutralized a free radical in the gut membrane, and it regenerates glutathione — the gut wall's primary antioxidant defense — from its oxidized form. The antioxidant network in the gut, as elsewhere, requires all of its members to function. Vitamin C cannot protect the gut membrane when vitamin E, glutathione, and selenium are depleted alongside it.

Phosphatidylcholine — The Mucus Layer's Hydrophobic Shield

The innermost mucus layer of the colon — the layer directly above the epithelial cells — is not merely a gel. It is a hydrophobic barrier whose water-repelling character is essential for keeping the luminal bacteria from penetrating to the epithelium below. This hydrophobic character is provided by phosphatidylcholine, which is present in high concentrations in the inner mucus layer and constitutes approximately seventy percent of its phospholipid content.

In ulcerative colitis — the inflammatory bowel disease that primarily affects the colon — phosphatidylcholine concentrations in the inner mucus layer are dramatically reduced, and the hydrophobic barrier function is impaired. Oral phosphatidylcholine supplementation has been shown in clinical trials to reduce disease activity in ulcerative colitis patients unresponsive to standard therapy, providing a nutrient-based intervention for a condition universally treated with immunosuppressants. This evidence is published, replicated, and essentially unknown in routine clinical practice.

Its essential partner: Phosphatidylcholine synthesis requires choline — a nutrient covered in the methylation cluster — and adequate methionine for the methyl groups required in the CDP-choline pathway. The gut's structural lipid integrity is therefore connected to the methylation network, demonstrating again how no cluster in this book operates in isolation from the others.

V. The Six Modern Assaults on the Gateway

The gut wall has been under sustained assault from six directions simultaneously since the mid-twentieth century — assaults that have no precedent in evolutionary history and whose cumulative effects the medical system has been extraordinarily slow to recognize.

Antibiotics — The Nuclear Option

A single course of broad-spectrum antibiotics reduces gut microbiome diversity by twenty to thirty percent and alters microbial composition in ways that may persist for months or years. In some individuals, the pre-antibiotic composition never fully recovers. Four courses, as Margaret received, represent four separate devastations of the ecosystem that produces butyrate, synthesizes vitamins, calibrates immune function, produces neurotransmitter precursors, and determines the bioavailability of every nutrient passing through the gut. The antibiotics were prescribed appropriately for acute infections. Their nutritional and microbiological aftermath was never considered or addressed.

Proton Pump Inhibitors — The Acid Suppression Paradox

Stomach acid serves functions beyond protein digestion. It sterilizes the stomach contents, preventing bacterial overgrowth in the upper gastrointestinal tract. It ionizes minerals — converting them from their food-bound forms to the free ionic forms that intestinal transporters recognize. It activates pepsin for protein digestion. And it provides the acid pH required to dissociate intrinsic factor from dietary vitamin B12 — the step without which

B12 cannot be absorbed. Suppressing stomach acid with proton pump inhibitors impairs all of these functions simultaneously. The nutrients that depend on adequate gastric acid for their absorption — magnesium, zinc, iron, B12, calcium, and thiamine — become less bioavailable regardless of dietary intake or supplementation. Margaret's three years on a proton pump inhibitor represent three years during which the most effective intervention for her deficiencies — correcting the acid environment that determines their absorption — was being pharmaceutically blocked.

Emulsifiers and Ultra-Processed Food

Dietary emulsifiers — carboxymethylcellulose and polysorbate 80, among the most commonly used — have been shown in animal studies to disrupt the mucus layer, alter gut microbiome composition, and increase intestinal permeability. Human studies have confirmed alterations in gut microbiome composition with emulsifier consumption. The Western diet provides emulsifiers in virtually every processed food product — breads, sauces, dairy alternatives, frozen meals, confectionery — at a frequency and quantity that has no ancestral precedent and whose cumulative effects on the gut wall are only beginning to be understood.

Chronic Stress — The Cortisol Connection

The gut and the brain communicate bidirectionally through the gut-brain axis. Chronic psychological stress activates the sympathetic nervous system and the hypothalamic-pituitary-adrenal axis, releasing cortisol and catecholamines that alter gut motility, reduce mucosal blood flow, increase gut permeability, and shift microbiome composition toward stress-associated patterns. The gut responds to the emotional state of the person it inhabits. A person under chronic stress has a more permeable gut wall, a more dysbiotic microbiome, and a less effective mucosal immune system — regardless of what they eat.

Chlorinated Water and Environmental Disruption

The chlorine added to municipal water supplies to kill pathogenic bacteria does not distinguish between pathogens and the commensal bacteria of the gut microbiome. Chronic exposure to chlorinated water suppresses beneficial bacterial populations over time. Combined with the antimicrobial compounds in hand soaps, cleaning products, and food preservatives, the modern environment constitutes a sustained low-level antimicrobial pressure on the gut microbiome that has no historical precedent.

Glyphosate — The Herbicide in the Food

Glyphosate — the active ingredient in the most widely used herbicide in the world — inhibits the shikimate pathway, a biochemical route used by bacteria (but not human cells) to synthesize aromatic amino acids. The gut microbiome, which contains trillions of bacteria, is therefore directly affected by dietary glyphosate exposure. Research has documented that glyphosate exposure reduces populations of beneficial bacteria including Lactobacillus and Bifidobacterium species while being relatively less toxic to opportunistic pathogens. The clinical implications of chronic low-level dietary glyphosate exposure on gut microbiome composition and function are only beginning to be characterized, but the biochemical mechanism of harm is clearly established.

VI. The Web of Dependencies

The gut gateway is not merely a passive recipient of the nutrients listed in this chapter. It is the structure through which every nutrient in every other chapter must pass before it can reach the cells that need it. This means that gut dysfunction is upstream of every other nutritional insufficiency in the book.

A person with a compromised gut wall absorbs less magnesium from their food — worsening the energy insufficiency described in Cluster 1. They absorb less zinc — weakening the immune system described in Cluster 8. They absorb less iron — impairing the structural scaffolding of the electron transport chain. They absorb less vitamin B12 — disrupting the methylation network of Cluster 9. The gut is not one cluster among equals. It is the prerequisite cluster. Everything else depends on it being functional first.

This dependency creates a treatment sequencing principle that standard medicine never explicitly articulates: when nutritional insufficiencies are identified and gut dysfunction is also present, addressing gut health is not an adjunct to nutritional restoration. It is the precondition for it. Supplementing nutrients into a dysfunctional gut is like pouring water into a bucket with holes — some gets in, but the throughput is a fraction of what it should be, and the bucket never fills.

> *The gut is the concert hall, the acoustics, and the ticket office simultaneously. Every musician in every cluster of this book must pass through it to reach their audience. When the hall is damaged, the performance suffers — not because the musicians are inadequate, but because the venue cannot deliver the sound.*

VII. Questions Worth Asking

For a person with persistent digestive symptoms, unexplained nutrient deficiencies that do not respond to supplementation, recurrent infections, skin conditions that wax and wane, mood instability, or fatigue that does not respond to thyroid management or iron repletion — the gut represents a compelling upstream territory that standard medical investigation rarely explores in depth.

Intestinal permeability can be assessed through urine lactulose-mannitol ratio testing — a non-invasive measure of paracellular gut barrier function. Comprehensive stool analysis can characterize microbiome composition, short-chain fatty acid production, secretory IgA levels, and markers of gut immune function. Calprotectin in stool indicates gut inflammation. Zonulin in serum — a protein that regulates tight junction opening — is elevated in increased permeability. None of these tests is on a standard panel.

None is routinely discussed at a primary care visit. All represent potentially valuable upstream information for anyone with the symptom picture described above.

> *The information in this chapter is presented to inform, not to prescribe. Gut health interventions — including dietary changes, probiotic use, and testing — should be undertaken in conversation with a qualified healthcare professional who can assess individual clinical context. The author is not a clinician and does not offer clinical advice.*

VIII. Margaret's Gateway, Reconsidered

Three years on a proton pump inhibitor. Four courses of broad-spectrum antibiotics. A decade of chronic stress. A processed-food diet rich in emulsifiers and low in the fermentable fiber that feeds butyrate-producing bacteria. A supplementation program that was delivering nutrients to a gateway that could not fully process them.

Margaret's gut was not failing at any single, diagnosable point. It was degrading across multiple dimensions simultaneously — thinning mucus from threonine and vitamin A insufficiency, loosening tight junctions from zinc depletion, producing less butyrate from a fiber-depleted and antibiotic-disrupted microbiome, absorbing minerals less effectively from acid suppression, and allowing a chronic background LPS leak that was contributing to the systemic inflammation that complicated her thyroid autoimmunity, her anxiety, and her skin condition.

None of this was on the map that medicine gave her. It was not diagnosed because medicine does not routinely investigate it. It was not treated because medicine does not routinely treat it with the tools that would be appropriate — dietary fiber, fermented foods, probiotic strains with documented evidence, glutamine, zinc, vitamin A, threonine, and a serious conversation about whether the proton pump inhibitor she had been taking for three years was still earning its place.

What Margaret needed was not a gastroenterologist. She needed a framework in which her gut was understood as the gateway through which every other intervention in her care either succeeded or failed. The framework exists. It simply was not part of the consultation she received.

For the Clinically Curious

Intestinal Permeability — Mechanisms and Measurement

Tight junction integrity is maintained by claudin and occludin proteins assembled around the scaffolding protein ZO-1 (zonula occludens-1). The opening of tight junctions is regulated by myosin light chain kinase (MLCK), which phosphorylates myosin and contracts the perijunctional actomyosin ring, pulling the tight junction apart. Inflammatory cytokines — particularly TNF-α and IFN-γ — upregulate MLCK expression, directly linking gut inflammation to increased permeability. The lactulose-mannitol urinary ratio test exploits differential permeability: mannitol crosses by transcellular transport and indicates villous surface area; lactulose crosses only paracellularly and indicates tight junction permeability. A ratio above 0.07 is generally considered indicative of increased permeability.

Zonulin — The Molecular Gatekeeper of Tight Junctions

Zonulin is a mammalian analogue of the Vibrio cholerae toxin ZOT that regulates the opening of intestinal tight junctions. Elevated serum zonulin correlates with increased intestinal permeability across a range of conditions including celiac disease, type 1 diabetes, multiple sclerosis, non-alcoholic fatty liver disease, and irritable bowel syndrome. Gliadin — the protein component of gluten — is a potent zonulin activator, providing a mechanistic basis for the gut permeability associated with gluten consumption in susceptible individuals independent of classical celiac autoimmunity. Serum zonulin testing is commercially available but not standardized; interpretation should account for pre-analytical variability.

LPS Endotoxemia — From Gut to Brain

Lipopolysaccharide (LPS) is a component of the outer membrane of gram-negative bacteria. It is recognized by Toll-like receptor 4 (TLR4) on macrophages and other immune cells, triggering NF-κB activation and inflammatory cytokine production. In conditions of increased gut permeability, LPS translocates from the gut lumen to the portal circulation and thence to the systemic circulation — a state termed metabolic endotoxemia. Systemic LPS concentrations two to three times above baseline have been documented in individuals consuming high-fat Western diets, activating TLR4 on circulating monocytes and on microglia in the brain. The resulting neuroinflammation provides a mechanistic link between gut dysbiosis, increased permeability, and conditions including depression, cognitive decline, and fatigue — conditions for which no gut investigation is currently standard of care.

Phosphatidylcholine and Ulcerative Colitis — Clinical Evidence

A randomized controlled trial published in Annals of Internal Medicine (Stremmel et al., 2005) demonstrated that modified-release oral phosphatidylcholine at 6g daily significantly reduced disease activity in patients with mild-to-moderate ulcerative colitis unresponsive to mesalazine. A subsequent phase II trial confirmed clinical remission rates significantly exceeding placebo. The proposed mechanism — restoration of the hydrophobic barrier function of the inner mucus layer — is consistent with the documented reduction in colonic phosphatidylcholine concentrations in ulcerative colitis patients compared to controls. This evidence base has not been translated into clinical guidelines despite its mechanistic plausibility and clinical documentation.

Butyrate — Epigenetic Mechanisms

Butyrate's anti-inflammatory and barrier-protective effects are mediated substantially through its activity as an inhibitor of class I and class IIb histone deacetylases (HDACs). HDAC inhibition maintains histones in their acetylated state, preserving the open chromatin configuration that enables expression of genes encoding tight junction proteins, anti-inflammatory cytokines, and anti-apoptotic factors in colonocytes.

Butyrate also activates free fatty acid receptor 2 (FFAR2) and FFAR3 on colonic L-cells, stimulating GLP-1 and PYY secretion, which suppress appetite and modulate glucose metabolism. The systemic metabolic effects of adequate butyrate production extend well beyond colonic mucosal health.

Cluster 3

The Garden Within

How the Trillions of Microorganisms That Share Your Body Determine Your Immunity, Your Mood, Your Metabolism — and Whether Every Nutrient in This Book Reaches the Cells That Need It

"Tell me what you eat, and I will tell you what you are."

— Jean Anthelme Brillat-Savarin, 1826 — a remark more microbiologically precise than he could have known

---

I. The Tenants Who Run the Building

Margaret's most recent gastroenterologist had scoped her twice in four years. Both times the colon appeared normal — no polyps, no inflammation, no visible pathology. She was told her gut was fine. The report was technically accurate and clinically misleading, because it described what the camera could see and nothing about what the camera could not.

Inside Margaret's colon, invisible to any endoscope, lived approximately 38 trillion microbial cells — bacteria, archaea, fungi, and viruses — constituting an ecosystem as complex as a rainforest and as sensitive to disruption. This ecosystem had been damaged in ways that no biopsy could reveal and no standard panel could measure: four courses of broad-spectrum antibiotics had periodically devastated it, the proton pump inhibitor had altered the gastric environment from which it is seeded, the processed-food diet had starved it of the fiber that feeds its most beneficial members, and a decade of chronic stress had shifted its composition through the cortisol-microbiome axis that nobody in her care team had been taught to ask about.

Her gut was fine. Her microbiome was not. And the difference between those two statements — one about what medicine can see, the other about what it cannot — is the subject of this chapter.

II. Meet the Cast

The microbiome is an ecosystem, not a list of individual actors. But certain key members and processes have been characterized well enough that they can be introduced individually before their collective story is told.

- **Bifidobacterium species** — The dominant bacteria of the healthy infant gut and a key regulatory species throughout life. They digest human milk oligosaccharides, produce short-chain fatty acids, support IgA production in the gut mucosa, and drive regulatory T-cell development. Among the first casualties of antibiotic treatment.

- **Lactobacillus species** — A diverse genus whose members produce lactic acid that acidifies the gut environment, inhibit pathogen colonization, support the gut-brain axis through GABA and serotonin precursor production, and maintain vaginal health. Strain-specific clinical evidence covers antibiotic-associated diarrhea, eczema prevention, and mood modulation.
- **Faecalibacterium prausnitzii** — Among the most abundant bacteria in the healthy adult gut and a primary producer of butyrate. Consistently reduced in inflammatory bowel disease, type 2 diabetes, obesity, and depression. Its abundance is one of the most reliable indicators of gut and systemic health.
- **Akkermansia muciniphila** — A mucus-degrading bacterium that paradoxically strengthens the gut barrier by stimulating mucus renewal. Reduced in metabolic syndrome, obesity, and type 2 diabetes. Inversely associated with cardiovascular risk. The subject of intense interest as a next-generation probiotic.
- **Roseburia intestinalis** — A major butyrate producer whose decline in Western diets correlates with the reduced butyrate production that drives colonic inflammation, impaired gut barrier function, and systemic metabolic consequences.
- **Dietary fiber** — The microbiome's primary food source — not a single compound but a family of plant-derived polysaccharides that different bacteria ferment differently. Diversity of fiber feeds diversity of bacteria.

- **Polyphenols** — Plant compounds found in berries, dark chocolate, green tea, olive oil, and red wine that are transformed by gut bacteria into biologically active metabolites. Feed Akkermansia and Bifidobacterium species selectively. Urolithin A — a polyphenol metabolite — activates mitophagy.
- **Short-chain fatty acids** — The metabolic products of bacterial fiber fermentation: butyrate, propionate, and acetate. Butyrate fuels the colon, suppresses inflammation, and tightens the gut barrier. Propionate modulates liver metabolism. Acetate travels to peripheral tissues and modulates appetite and immunity.
- **Tryptophan** — Dietary amino acid whose metabolic fate in the gut is determined by microbial composition: toward serotonin (beneficial), toward kynurenine (inflammatory, potentially neurotoxic), or toward protective indole metabolites depending on which bacteria are present.
- **The vagus nerve** — The primary bidirectional highway of the gut-brain axis, carrying signals from gut microbiome and enteric nervous system to brain and from brain to gut. The physical channel through which the microbiome speaks to the mind.

These are the principal players. Together they constitute an ecosystem whose disruption medicine has spent a century calling a gastrointestinal problem, and whose restoration may be the most consequential single intervention available for a wide spectrum of conditions that standard care has treated as having nothing to do with the gut.

III. What the Microbiome Actually Does

Nutrient Synthesis and Bioavailability

The gut microbiome synthesizes vitamin K2 — the menaquinone forms that direct calcium into bone and away from arterial walls. It produces biotin and contributes to the availability of other B vitamins. It converts dietary folate from polyglutamate forms to the absorbable monoglutamate form. And through fermentation, it produces the short-chain fatty acids that acidify the distal intestine, improving calcium, magnesium, and iron absorption in the colon.

Perhaps most remarkably, the microbiome determines the bioavailability of dietary polyphenols — plant compounds that appear in food in forms that human digestive enzymes cannot convert to their active metabolites. Ellagitannins in pomegranate and walnuts are converted by gut bacteria to urolithins only in individuals harboring the right bacterial species. Quercetin, resveratrol, and curcumin are similarly transformed by gut bacteria into more bioavailable and more biologically active forms. The nutritional value of polyphenol-rich foods is not fixed — it is a function of the microbial community that processes them.

Immune Education — The Microbial School

Seventy percent of the body's immune tissue lines the gut. This is not anatomical coincidence. The gut is where the immune system receives its primary education in distinguishing self from non-self, pathogen from commensal, danger from tolerance. From the first hours of life — when the newborn's gut is colonized by maternal and environmental bacteria — the immune system is being programmed by its microbial curriculum.

Regulatory T cells — the immune system's internal governors, responsible for preventing excessive inflammatory responses and autoimmune attack — are produced in large numbers in the gut-associated lymphoid tissue under the instruction of specific bacterial species including certain Clostridia and Bifidobacterium strains, and their development depends on short-chain fatty acid signaling from butyrate. Children who receive multiple antibiotic courses during the critical first three years of immune programming show higher rates of allergic and autoimmune conditions in later childhood — not because the antibiotics directly caused these conditions, but because the microbiome disruption they produced impaired the immune education that would have prevented them.

The Gut-Brain Axis — Ninety Percent of Serotonin

Approximately ninety percent of the body's serotonin is produced in the gut — not the brain. Enterochromaffin cells in the intestinal epithelium synthesize serotonin under the direct stimulation of specific gut bacterial species, particularly Clostridia and spore-forming bacteria of the Lachnospiraceae family. This gut-derived serotonin does not cross the blood-brain barrier and does not directly affect mood — but it is central to gut motility regulation, and its production is intimately connected to the gut-brain signaling that does affect mood through vagal and endocrine pathways.

The gut produces not only serotonin precursors but GABA directly, and modulates the GABAergic system through vagal signaling. Lactobacillus rhamnosus JB-1 — in animal studies that remain the basis for subsequent human research — directly influences GABA receptor expression in the brain through vagal signaling, reducing anxiety and depressive behavior. This finding spawned the concept of the psychobiotic — a probiotic strain with specific neuro-modulatory effects — and a research field that is rapidly accumulating human clinical evidence.

The implications for psychiatry are profound and largely unacknowledged in clinical practice. A patient treated for anxiety or depression with pharmaceutical manipulation of central serotonin or GABA systems, whose gut microbiome has been repeatedly devastated by antibiotics and depleted by a low-fiber diet, is having their downstream symptoms addressed while the upstream dysregulation continues. The brain chemistry being pharmaceutically managed is a downstream expression of gut ecology.

> *Ninety percent of the serotonin in the human body is made in the gut. Every prescription for an SSRI — a drug designed to increase serotonin availability in the brain — is written without a single question about the health of the ecosystem that produces the majority of the*

> *body's serotonin. The upstream goes uninvestigated. The downstream gets medicated. The pattern is the same.*

IV. The Six Modern Assaults

The gut barrier chapter detailed how antibiotics, proton pump inhibitors, processed food, chronic stress, and environmental chemicals compromise the physical gateway. The same five forces strike the ecosystem that gateway protects — with consequences distinct enough to warrant their own accounting, and a sixth assault that begins before a person's first meal.

Antibiotics — Beyond the Physical Barrier

A single course of broad-spectrum antibiotics can eliminate more than one-third of gut bacterial species within days, and certain species fail to return to pre-treatment abundance even six months later. The four courses Margaret received represent four separate ecological crises. Children average ten antibiotic courses by age ten — each one striking during the critical window when the microbiome is still programming the immune system's lifelong tolerance and reactivity settings.

Proton Pump Inhibitors — Beyond Mineral Absorption

The same acid suppression that blocks mineral uptake removes the chemical barrier that keeps bacteria from colonizing the small intestine, producing small intestinal bacterial overgrowth — a measurable consequence beyond the absorption failure already described.

Processed Food — Starving the Ecosystem

The Western diet provides roughly fifteen grams of fiber daily against an ancestral baseline of fifty to one hundred. The bacteria most associated with gut health — Faecalibacterium prausnitzii, Roseburia intestinalis, Bifidobacterium — are fiber fermenters first. Starved of their food supply, they decline regardless of how intact the physical barrier remains.

Chronic Stress — The Bidirectional Trap

Cortisol reshapes microbiome composition toward inflammatory patterns; a disrupted microbiome in turn heightens cortisol reactivity to stress. Medicating either side of this loop alone leaves the other intact.

Glyphosate — The Shikimate Pathway

Glyphosate inhibits a biochemical pathway bacteria use to synthesize tryptophan — the precursor for serotonin — without affecting human cells directly, which lack this pathway. The mechanism is sound; the evidence at typical dietary exposure remains emerging.

Birth and Early Life — The First Seeding

The microbiome's founding population is set at birth. Vaginally delivered infants inherit it from the birth canal; cesarean-delivered infants inherit a skin-dominant microbiome whose differences persist for years and correlate with higher rates of allergic disease, asthma, and obesity. Breast milk's human milk oligosaccharides — indigestible to the infant directly — exist for the sole purpose of feeding Bifidobacterium. Formula cannot replicate them. This is the one assault that begins before any of the other five have a chance to act.

V. The Gut-Brain Axis in Clinical Practice

The gut-brain axis is bidirectional — signals travel from gut to brain and from brain to gut with equal importance. The physical channels include the vagus nerve (carrying sensory information from the gut to the brainstem), the enteric nervous system (the 500-million-neuron nervous system of the gut that operates semi-independently), the portal circulation (through which gut-derived metabolites and inflammatory signals reach the liver and systemic circulation), and the endocrine system (through which gut hormones — GLP-1, PYY, ghrelin, CCK — communicate satiety, glucose status, and stress signals to the brain).

Clinical conditions that are now understood through the gut-brain axis include irritable bowel syndrome (visceral hypersensitivity and altered gut motility driven by enteric nervous system sensitization and microbiome dysbiosis), major depression (consistently associated with reduced gut microbiome diversity, reduced Lactobacillus and Bifidobacterium populations, elevated systemic LPS from increased gut permeability, and elevated kynurenine pathway metabolites that compete with tryptophan for brain entry), anxiety (bidirectionally linked with gut dysbiosis in both animal and human studies), Alzheimer's disease (associated with specific microbiome compositional patterns and elevated gut-derived amyloid from oral and gut bacteria), and Parkinson's disease (now understood to potentially begin in the gut, with enteric nervous system Lewy body pathology preceding central nervous system involvement by years in some patients).

The clinical implications are both sobering and actionable. A patient treated for depression with antidepressants alone, whose gut microbiome has been repeatedly disrupted by antibiotics and depleted by a low-fiber processed-food diet, is being treated at the downstream end of a system whose upstream cause is structural and addressable. The antidepressant may help. But the microbiome disruption continues, the gut permeability continues, the systemic LPS-mediated neuroinflammation continues, and the tryptophan diversion through the kynurenine pathway continues — none of it visible to the prescribing psychiatrist, none of it addressed by the serotonin reuptake inhibitor in the prescription.

VI. Leaky Gut — When the Barrier Fails

The term leaky gut has been treated by mainstream medicine as an alternative health concept without clinical substance. The science does not support this dismissal. Increased intestinal permeability is a measurable, reproducible physiological state that can be quantified by lactulose-mannitol ratio testing, tight junction protein assays, and serum markers of bacterial translocation, and whose association with systemic inflammatory disease is documented across a large and growing literature.

When the intestinal barrier is disrupted — by dysbiosis, by dietary emulsifiers damaging the mucus layer, by psychological stress, by alcohol, or by NSAIDs — the normally selective barrier becomes non-selective. Bacterial lipopolysaccharide translocates from the gut lumen into the systemic circulation, producing metabolic endotoxemia: a low-grade chronic inflammatory activation now mechanistically linked to insulin resistance, metabolic syndrome, cardiovascular disease, neuroinflammation, and depression. Serum zonulin — a protein that regulates tight junction opening — is elevated in conditions ranging from celiac disease to multiple sclerosis, type 1 diabetes, autism spectrum disorder, and Parkinson's disease, suggesting that gut barrier disruption is a common upstream feature of diseases whose apparent unifying thread is inflammation.

> *The conditions most consistently associated with elevated serum zonulin span the specialties that medicine has organized into separate silos: rheumatoid arthritis, fibromyalgia, chronic fatigue syndrome, depression, anxiety, Hashimoto's thyroiditis. These are not coincidentally clustered. They are different expressions of a common upstream state — intestinal hyperpermeability driving systemic inflammatory activation — that has been labeled differently by the specialty that first encountered each downstream manifestation.*

VII. Restoring the Garden

Microbiome restoration is not a product. It is a process. No single probiotic supplement can restore a damaged microbial ecosystem in the absence of the dietary, lifestyle, and environmental changes that created the damage. The restoration process has a logical sequence: reduce the ongoing disruptors, reintroduce beneficial species, and sustain them with the dietary conditions they need to thrive.

Feeding Diversity

The number of different plant species consumed per week is the strongest dietary predictor of gut microbiome diversity in large population studies, including the American Gut Project. Thirty or more different plant foods per week — different vegetables, fruits, legumes, whole grains, nuts, seeds, herbs, and spices — is associated with significantly greater microbial diversity than diets providing fewer than ten species. Every different plant food provides a different fiber substrate for a different bacterial community. The instruction is elegant in its simplicity: eat more different plants.

Fermented Foods — Live Cultures and Metabolic Products

A 2021 Stanford randomized controlled trial directly compared a high-fermented-food diet with a high-fiber diet in healthy adults. The fermented food group — consuming yogurt, kefir, fermented cottage cheese, kimchi, sauerkraut, and kombucha — showed significantly increased microbiome diversity and significantly reduced systemic inflammatory markers at ten weeks. The high-fiber group showed neither improvement, possibly because the fiber was being consumed by an ecosystem that lacked the diversity to ferment it efficiently. The finding suggests that for individuals with already-depleted microbial diversity, introducing live microbial cultures alongside their prebiotic food may be more effective than increasing fiber alone.

Targeted Probiotic Support

Strain specificity is the critical principle. Lactobacillus rhamnosus GG has the strongest evidence for antibiotic-associated diarrhea prevention and treatment in children. Saccharomyces boulardii has strong evidence for C. difficile-associated diarrhea and traveler's diarrhea in adults. Bifidobacterium longum 1714 has emerging evidence for anxiety and stress response modulation. Multi-strain products providing both Lactobacillus and Bifidobacterium species are appropriate for general microbiome maintenance support. The appropriate strain, dose, and duration for any specific clinical indication is a clinical determination requiring professional guidance.

VIII. Questions Worth Asking

For a person with persistent digestive symptoms, recurrent infections, mood instability, fatigue, skin conditions, or nutrient deficiencies that do not respond to supplementation — the microbiome represents territory that standard medical investigation essentially never explores in depth.

Comprehensive stool analysis can characterize microbiome composition, short-chain fatty acid production, secretory IgA levels, and markers of gut immune function. Serum zonulin and LPS-binding protein provide systemic markers of gut barrier integrity. Breath testing for hydrogen and methane measures bacterial fermentation in the small intestine (SIBO assessment). None of these tests are on a standard panel. None are routinely offered at a primary care visit. All represent potentially valuable upstream information for anyone whose clinical picture includes the multi-system involvement that gut dysbiosis and increased permeability are now documented to produce.

The information in this chapter is educational and does not constitute clinical advice. Microbiome testing and any interventions based on it should be discussed with a qualified healthcare professional. Probiotic use in immunocompromised individuals requires medical supervision. Specific probiotic strains mentioned in this chapter are referenced as examples of strain-specific evidence and do not constitute recommendations for any individual's use without appropriate professional assessment.

IX. Margaret's Garden, Reconsidered

Four antibiotic courses. Three years on a proton pump inhibitor. A processed-food diet providing approximately fifteen grams of fiber daily and regular exposure to emulsifiers. A decade of chronic stress. No fermented foods. No assessment of microbiome function. No conversation about gut health beyond the endoscopy that found nothing wrong.

Margaret's gut camera saw a normal colon. What it could not see was a microbiome that had been repeatedly devastated and never properly restored, producing less butyrate than her colonic epithelium needed, delivering less serotonin precursor to her enterochromaffin cells than her anxiety-prone nervous system required, allowing more LPS into her systemic circulation than her chronically activated immune system needed to remain calm, and synthesizing less vitamin K2 than her cardiovascular system needed to direct calcium properly.

The conventional scope found nothing wrong. The unconventional questions — about diversity, about fiber, about the four antibiotic courses, about what happens to a microbiome that has been repeatedly disrupted and never systematically restored — were never asked. The garden was failing in silence while the camera panned its surfaces and declared them intact.

For the Clinically Curious

The Tryptophan-Kynurenine-Serotonin Triad

Dietary tryptophan is metabolized through two major competing pathways: the serotonin pathway (tryptophan → 5-HTP → serotonin → melatonin) and the kynurenine pathway (tryptophan → kynurenine → quinolinic acid or kynurenic acid). Under conditions of systemic inflammation — including the LPS-mediated inflammatory activation of gut dysbiosis — indoleamine 2,3-dioxygenase (IDO) is upregulated, diverting tryptophan preferentially into the kynurenine pathway. Quinolinic acid, a downstream kynurenine metabolite, is an NMDA receptor agonist with neurotoxic properties at elevated concentrations, and is consistently elevated in depression. The IDO-mediated tryptophan diversion toward quinolinic acid provides a mechanistic connection between gut dysbiosis, systemic inflammation, reduced serotonin precursor availability, and depression that the psychiatry literature is only beginning to integrate.

Akkermansia muciniphila — Next-Generation Probiotic

Akkermansia muciniphila is a gram-negative, strictly anaerobic bacterium that resides in the mucus layer of the gut and constitutes approximately one to three percent of the healthy adult microbiome. Its abundance is inversely correlated with obesity, metabolic syndrome, type 2 diabetes, inflammatory bowel disease, and cardiovascular disease in multiple population studies. The mechanism involves Amuc_1100 — a bacterial outer membrane protein that activates TLR2 signaling in intestinal epithelial cells, enhancing tight junction expression and improving gut barrier function. Pasteurized A.

muciniphila (inactivated but not killed) has been shown in a human randomized controlled trial to improve insulin sensitivity and reduce cardiometabolic risk markers at three months, potentially with superior efficacy to the live form due to greater stability. A. muciniphila is now available as a commercial supplement in some markets, though regulatory status varies by jurisdiction.

Short-Chain Fatty Acids — Systemic Metabolic Effects

Propionate — produced by Bacteroidetes fermentation of certain fibers — travels to the liver through the portal circulation, where it inhibits cholesterol synthesis (via HMG-CoA reductase), gluconeogenesis, and de novo lipogenesis while enhancing insulin sensitivity. These hepatic effects of colonic bacterial fermentation products represent a mechanism by which dietary fiber directly modulates lipid and glucose metabolism — a mechanism absent from the pharmacological model of cardiovascular and metabolic disease management. Acetate circulates systemically and activates FFAR2 on adipocytes and immune cells, modulating adipogenesis and macrophage inflammatory state. The systemic reach of butyrate, propionate, and acetate from colonic fermentation — cardiovascular, metabolic, immunological, neurological — represents one of the strongest arguments for viewing dietary fiber as a systemic therapeutic rather than simply a digestive aid.

Urolithins — Mitophagy Activation Through the Microbiome

Urolithin A is produced by the gut bacterial metabolism of ellagitannins from pomegranate, walnuts, strawberries, and raspberries. Only approximately forty percent of Western adults harbor the specific bacterial species — Gordonibacter urolithinfaciens and Ellagibacter isourolithinifaciens among them — required for urolithin A production, explaining why ellagitannin-rich foods produce markedly different biological effects in different individuals. Urolithin A activates mitophagy through PINK1/Parkin signaling and PGC-1α upregulation, clearing damaged mitochondria and promoting mitochondrial biogenesis. A phase I human trial demonstrated that urolithin A supplementation improved skeletal muscle mitochondrial function, reduced inflammatory markers, and improved physical performance — connecting microbiome-mediated postbiotic production to mitochondrial health with direct clinical evidence.

Cluster 4

The Antioxidant Shield

How Eight Nutrients Protect Every Cell From the Combustion Products of Being Alive — and What Happens When the Shield Develops Holes

> *"We are oxidative creatures. We breathe oxygen, we burn fuel, and in doing so we generate fire. The question is not whether we oxidize — we do. The question is whether we have the means to contain the fire."*

I. The Fire Inside

Consider David. He is forty-seven years old, a software engineer who has never smoked, runs three miles twice a week, and takes a daily multivitamin that he has selected based on the label's promise of antioxidant support. His last physical found nothing remarkable. His cholesterol is borderline, his inflammatory markers are at the upper end of normal, and he has noticed over the past two years that he recovers more slowly from exercise than he used to. He bruises more easily. A small cut on his hand took three weeks to heal fully, rather than the usual ten days. His energy in the afternoons has become unreliable.

David's story is not dramatic. It does not involve a crisis, a diagnosis, or a specialist referral. It involves something quieter and in some ways more consequential: the slow accumulation of oxidative damage in cells that are not being adequately protected from the combustion products of their own metabolism.

Every cell in the human body burns fuel to produce energy. The burning is not metaphorical. The electron transport chain — described in Cluster 1 — is a controlled combustion process, and like all combustion processes, it generates reactive byproducts. The primary byproduct is superoxide — an oxygen molecule that has accepted one extra electron and become chemically unstable, seeking a molecular partner with which to react. Superoxide reacts with whatever is nearest: the lipids of the cell membrane, the proteins of the mitochondrial wall, the DNA in the cell's nucleus. The damage it causes is cumulative, structural, and — without adequate antioxidant defense — irreversible.

The antioxidant defense system is the body's method for containing this fire. It is not one molecule or one enzyme. It is a network of eight nutrients working in precise coordination, each neutralizing specific reactive species at specific locations, each regenerating the others after they have been used, each dependent on the rest of the network to function. Remove one member of this network and the fire spreads further before it is contained. Remove several and the fire begins to win.

II. Meet the Cast

Eight musicians comprise the antioxidant orchestra described in this chapter. Together they cover the full range of cellular compartments — from the water-soluble interior of the cell to the fat-soluble membranes of the mitochondria — and from the primary neutralization of reactive oxygen species to the regeneration of the network itself.

- **Selenium** — The mineral at the center of glutathione peroxidase — the body's primary enzyme for neutralizing hydrogen peroxide, one of the most damaging reactive oxygen species. Also the cofactor for thioredoxin reductase, the second major branch of the antioxidant enzyme system.
- **Vitamin C** — The water-soluble primary antioxidant that neutralizes reactive species in the aqueous environment of the cell interior and bloodstream. After neutralizing a free radical, it becomes dehydroascorbate — and is then regenerated by glutathione, making it dependent on the entire downstream network.
- **Vitamin E (tocopherols and tocotrienols)** — The fat-soluble antioxidant that neutralizes lipid peroxyl radicals in cell membranes and the inner mitochondrial membrane — precisely where the electron transport chain operates and where oxidative damage is most consequential. After

neutralizing a radical, vitamin E becomes a tocopheroxyl radical and is regenerated by vitamin C.

- **Copper** — As the mineral at the center of copper-zinc superoxide dismutase (Cu/Zn-SOD), copper neutralizes superoxide in the cytoplasm — the cell's first line of defense against the primary reactive oxygen species generated by metabolism.
- **Zinc** — Partners with copper in Cu/Zn-SOD, stabilizing the enzyme's structure and completing the active site. Also present in zinc-finger antioxidant proteins that protect DNA from oxidative damage.
- **Manganese** — The mineral at the center of manganese superoxide dismutase (MnSOD) — the mitochondria's internal antioxidant enzyme. While Cu/Zn-SOD operates in the cytoplasm, MnSOD operates inside the mitochondrial matrix, at the site of primary superoxide generation.
- **Glutathione** — The body's master antioxidant molecule — a tripeptide of glutamate, cysteine, and glycine that neutralizes hydrogen peroxide (via glutathione peroxidase), regenerates vitamin C from dehydroascorbate, and detoxifies reactive metabolites in the liver. The hub around which the entire antioxidant network rotates.
- **Alpha-lipoic acid** — The only antioxidant that operates in both water-soluble and fat-soluble environments, and the only one capable of regenerating glutathione, vitamin C, and vitamin E simultaneously. The antioxidant network's reset button.

These eight musicians are not independent soloists. They are a system, and the system has directionality: primary neutralization, then radical handoff, then regeneration, then recycling. Each step requires a different player. Remove any one, and the cascade stalls at that point.

III. How the Shield Works — A Map for the General Reader

The antioxidant defense system can be understood through a simple sequence: generation, neutralization, regeneration, and recycling. Understanding this sequence transforms the list of eight nutrients from a catalogue into a story.

Generation — Where the Fire Starts

The electron transport chain, while producing ATP, generates superoxide as a byproduct when electrons leak from Complexes I and III before reaching their intended destination. This is not a malfunction. It is an inevitable consequence of high-speed electron transfer. Under normal conditions, approximately one to three percent of the oxygen consumed by mitochondria becomes superoxide rather than water. The mitochondrion produces approximately 10 billion ATP molecules per second per cell — meaning the generation of reactive oxygen species is continuous, massive, and unavoidable.

First Response — MnSOD and Cu/Zn-SOD

Superoxide's first encounter is with superoxide dismutase. Inside the mitochondria, MnSOD — whose active site contains manganese — converts superoxide to hydrogen peroxide. In the cytoplasm just outside the mitochondria, Cu/Zn-SOD — whose active site contains both copper and zinc — performs the same conversion. The reaction is: two superoxide molecules + two hydrogen ions → hydrogen peroxide + oxygen. Hydrogen peroxide is less reactive than superoxide but still dangerous — particularly because it can react with iron to form the hydroxyl radical, which is among the most destructive reactive species known to biology.

Second Response — Glutathione Peroxidase

Hydrogen peroxide is neutralized by glutathione peroxidase — a selenium-containing enzyme that converts hydrogen peroxide to water using glutathione as the reducing agent. The reaction: hydrogen peroxide + 2 glutathione (reduced) → 2 water + glutathione disulfide (oxidized). After this reaction, glutathione is in its oxidized form and cannot neutralize another molecule of hydrogen peroxide until it is regenerated.

Regeneration — The Network Maintains Itself

Oxidized glutathione is regenerated to its reduced form by glutathione reductase, an enzyme that requires riboflavin (FAD) and niacin (NADPH). This is the connection between the antioxidant system and the energy-producing nutrients of Cluster 1: NADPH, derived from niacin through the pentose phosphate pathway, is the reducing agent that regenerates glutathione. Deplete niacin, and glutathione recycling falters. Deplete riboflavin, and it falters further.

Meanwhile, vitamin C regenerates vitamin E after it has neutralized a lipid peroxyl radical in the membrane. Glutathione regenerates vitamin C after it has given away its electrons. Alpha-lipoic acid can regenerate glutathione, vitamin C, and vitamin E simultaneously, operating as a master recycler that keeps the entire network running. The cascade has a direction: vitamin E → vitamin C → glutathione → glutathione reductase (riboflavin + NADPH) → back to active glutathione. Each link in this chain must be intact for the fire to be fully contained.

> *The antioxidant orchestra is the most interdependent section in the entire symphony. Every musician depends on the one before and the one after. When David's afternoon energy fails, when his wounds heal slowly, when his bruises persist longer than they should, the orchestra is not playing at full volume. The fire is spreading further than it should before being contained. And nobody has looked at the orchestra.*

IV. The Musicians, One by One

Selenium — The Peroxide Neutralizer

Selenium is a trace mineral whose biological function is almost entirely mediated through selenoproteins — a family of twenty-five proteins in which selenium is incorporated into the active site in the form of selenocysteine. The two most important for antioxidant defense are glutathione peroxidase, which neutralizes hydrogen peroxide and lipid hydroperoxides, and thioredoxin reductase, which reduces thioredoxin — a protein that itself regulates multiple redox-sensitive transcription factors and DNA repair enzymes.

Selenium deficiency produces a specific and striking clinical syndrome — Keshan disease, a cardiomyopathy affecting populations in selenium-poor soil regions of China — that is the most dramatic demonstration of selenium's essential cardiac role. Less dramatically but no less importantly, selenium insufficiency impairs the continuous neutralization of hydrogen peroxide that protects all tissues from oxidative damage: the brain, the thyroid, the gonads, and the cardiovascular system particularly.

The thyroid connection deserves emphasis: deiodinase enzymes, which convert the inactive thyroid hormone T4 to the active T3, are selenoproteins. Selenium deficiency therefore impairs thyroid hormone activation even when iodine and TSH are normal — a connection that explains why some patients on levothyroxine continue to feel hypothyroid despite apparently adequate T4 levels. Their selenium status was never checked.

Its essential partners: *Selenium works with vitamin E in the neutralization of lipid hydroperoxides — selenium handles the peroxide, vitamin E handles the membrane lipid radical that generates it. They are synergistic: selenium deficiency increases vitamin E requirements, and vice versa. Selenium also depends on adequate glutathione substrate — glutamine, cysteine, and glycine — for the glutathione peroxidase reaction to proceed.*

Vitamin C — The Water-Soluble Guardian

Vitamin C — ascorbic acid — is the premier water-soluble antioxidant in human biology, and the human requirement for it is a consequence of a mutation that inactivated the enzyme (L-gulonolactone oxidase) required to synthesize it from glucose. Most mammals make their own vitamin C; humans, other primates, guinea pigs, and a handful of other species must obtain it from food. The evolutionary implication is that the diet of our ancestors was sufficiently rich in ascorbate-containing foods that the gene for its synthesis became redundant. The modern diet, dominated by processed foods depleted of their vitamin C content by heat, oxidation, and storage, frequently is not.

Vitamin C neutralizes superoxide, hydrogen peroxide, hydroxyl radicals, singlet oxygen, and hypochlorite — covering virtually the full spectrum of reactive oxygen species generated by metabolic activity and immune function. It is also the cofactor for prolyl hydroxylase and lysyl hydroxylase, the enzymes that mature collagen — explaining why vitamin C deficiency produces the connective tissue failure of scurvy, and why subclinical insufficiency produces the bleeding gums, slow wound healing, and arterial wall fragility that Margaret experienced.

Linus Pauling's advocacy for high-dose vitamin C was controversial and remains partially unresolved. What is not controversial is that the RDA for vitamin C — established to prevent scurvy — bears no relationship to the doses required for optimal antioxidant defense, immune function, or collagen synthesis. The RDA prevents the historical deficiency disease. Optimal antioxidant status requires meaningfully higher intake, particularly under conditions of oxidative stress, illness, or smoking.

Its essential partners: *Vitamin C is regenerated by glutathione after neutralizing a free radical — meaning vitamin C's effectiveness as an antioxidant depends on adequate glutathione supply. When glutathione is depleted, vitamin C cannot be recycled and is consumed irreversibly. Alpha-lipoic acid regenerates vitamin C independently of glutathione, providing a backup recycling pathway. Vitamin C also enhances iron absorption — a double-edged function, valuable for iron deficiency but potentially problematic in iron overload.*

Vitamin E — The Membrane Guardian

The cell membrane and the inner mitochondrial membrane are composed of phospholipids — fat molecules whose polyunsaturated fatty acid tails are highly vulnerable to oxidative attack. When a free radical attacks a membrane fatty acid, it initiates a chain reaction called lipid peroxidation, in which each damaged fatty acid generates a new radical that attacks the next molecule, propagating damage through the membrane like a fire spreading through dry grass.

Vitamin E — specifically alpha-tocopherol, the primary tocopherol in human tissue — resides within the cell membrane, positioned to intercept lipid peroxyl radicals before they can initiate chain reactions. It donates a hydrogen atom to the radical, quenching it, and becomes itself a less reactive tocopheroxyl radical that is then regenerated by vitamin C.

The tocotrienol forms of vitamin E — found in palm oil, rice bran, and annatto — have structural differences that allow them to move more freely within membranes and may provide superior neuroprotective and anti-cancer properties relative to tocopherols. Most vitamin E research and supplementation has focused on alpha-tocopherol; the tocotrienols represent a more recently characterized and clinically underinvestigated aspect of vitamin E biology.

Its essential partner: *Vitamin E depends on vitamin C for its regeneration. This means that the membrane antioxidant system and the aqueous antioxidant system are coupled: vitamin E cannot continuously protect membranes unless vitamin C is available to regenerate it, and vitamin C cannot continuously operate unless glutathione is available to regenerate it. The network is a chain, and every link must hold.*

Copper and Zinc in SOD — The First Responders

Cu/Zn-SOD — the cytoplasmic superoxide dismutase — is a homodimer: two identical protein subunits, each containing one copper atom and one zinc atom at its active site. The copper cycles between its two oxidation states to dismutate superoxide. The zinc contributes structural stability to the active site rather than catalytic activity directly, but without it the enzyme does not fold correctly and cannot function.

The clinical importance of Cu/Zn-SOD extends beyond antioxidant defense into neurology: mutations in the gene encoding Cu/Zn-SOD are found in approximately twenty percent of familial amyotrophic lateral sclerosis (ALS) cases, and the resulting gain-of-toxic-function suggests that oxidative stress mediated through dysfunctional SOD is directly involved in motor neurone death. The nutrient that sits at the active site of this enzyme is copper — invisible to standard laboratory panels, rarely measured, almost never considered in the neurology clinic.

Its essential partners: *Copper and zinc must be in appropriate balance — not just adequately present individually. High-dose zinc supplementation suppresses copper absorption, and a zinc-copper imbalance can impair Cu/Zn-SOD function even when total enzyme protein is adequate. The ratio matters as much as the absolute amounts.*

Manganese — The Mitochondria's Internal Guard

MnSOD — manganese superoxide dismutase — sits inside the mitochondrial matrix, at the primary site of superoxide generation.

It is the first line of defense against the reactive oxygen species produced by the electron transport chain itself. Without adequate manganese, MnSOD cannot function, and the mitochondrion — already generating significant superoxide as a normal metabolic byproduct — has no internal defense.

The SOD2 gene encoding MnSOD has a well-studied variant — Val16Ala — that reduces the enzyme's import into the mitochondria and therefore its activity. Individuals with this variant have reduced mitochondrial antioxidant defense at baseline and are more vulnerable to oxidative damage under conditions of inadequate manganese. This is the genetic-nutritional interaction that Bruce Ames's triage theory predicted: a genetic variant that narrows the margin for nutritional sufficiency. The genetic test for SOD2 Val16Ala is available and increasingly used in functional medicine; the manganese status that determines the clinical significance of the variant is almost never measured.

Its essential partner: *Manganese shares intestinal absorption pathways with iron, and high iron intake suppresses manganese absorption. In populations eating high-iron diets or taking iron supplements, manganese status may be inadvertently compromised — yet another example of mineral competition whose clinical consequences are unmeasured.*

Glutathione — The Hub

Glutathione — gamma-glutamylcysteinylglycine — is the body's most abundant intracellular antioxidant and the hub around which the antioxidant network rotates. It consists of three amino acids:

glutamate, cysteine, and glycine. Cysteine is considered rate-limiting for its synthesis; glycine is equally important but less discussed. The liver is the primary site of glutathione synthesis and its primary storage organ.

Glutathione's functions extend well beyond antioxidant defense. It is the primary substrate for phase II liver detoxification — conjugating reactive metabolites for urinary or biliary excretion. It regulates immune cell function — T-cells require adequate intracellular glutathione to proliferate and respond to antigens. It modulates the activity of redox-sensitive transcription factors including NF-κB. And it directly neutralizes methylglyoxal — a toxic byproduct of glucose metabolism that accumulates in diabetes and contributes to diabetic complications.

Glutathione cannot be directly supplemented effectively because it is rapidly degraded in the gastrointestinal tract. The strategies for raising intracellular glutathione levels are to supplement its precursors — particularly N-acetylcysteine (NAC) for cysteine, and glycine, whose clinical depletion is underappreciated. A study published in Clinical Nutrition demonstrated that elderly individuals supplemented with NAC and glycine — but not either alone — restored glutathione levels to those of young adults and significantly improved markers of oxidative stress, insulin resistance, and mitochondrial function.

Its essential partners: *Glutathione requires riboflavin (as FAD) and niacin (as NADPH) for its regeneration by glutathione reductase. It requires selenium for the glutathione peroxidase* *reaction. It requires vitamin C as a partner in the antioxidant regeneration cascade. And it requires adequate glycine, cysteine, and glutamate as its structural building blocks. Glutathione is the hub precisely because so many other antioxidant nutrients feed into it or depend on it.*

Alpha-Lipoic Acid — The Network's Reset Button

Alpha-lipoic acid is unique in the antioxidant network for two properties that no other antioxidant possesses simultaneously: it is both fat-soluble and water-soluble, allowing it to operate in cell membranes and in the aqueous cell interior; and it can regenerate glutathione, vitamin C, and vitamin E, making it the only known molecule capable of recycling all three primary antioxidants.

Alpha-lipoic acid also functions as a cofactor for the pyruvate dehydrogenase complex and alpha-ketoglutarate dehydrogenase in the Krebs cycle — connecting it directly to the energy-producing network of Cluster 1. It chelates heavy metals including mercury, arsenic, and cadmium, and may play a role in their elimination. And its reduced form, dihydrolipoic acid, can regenerate coenzyme Q10 — the mobile electron carrier — from its oxidized ubiquinone form back to the antioxidant ubiquinol.

The body synthesizes alpha-lipoic acid, but production declines with age and under conditions of metabolic stress. Dietary sources — organ meats, red meat, and some vegetables — provide modest amounts. Supplemental alpha-lipoic acid is well-absorbed and has demonstrated clinical benefits in diabetic neuropathy, liver disease, and age-related cognitive decline — applications that reflect its multi-system antioxidant and metabolic roles.

Its essential partner: *Alpha-lipoic acid is most effective when adequate glutathione, vitamin C, and vitamin E are available — it regenerates all three, but it cannot regenerate them if they are absent. The reset button works only if there is something to reset.*

V. What Oxidative Stress Actually Produces

Understanding the antioxidant network becomes more urgent when the consequences of its insufficiency are made explicit. Oxidative stress is not a laboratory abstraction. It is a mechanism through which inadequate antioxidant defense produces specific, named, diagnosable diseases — diseases that medicine treats at their downstream manifestations while the upstream fire continues burning.

Cardiovascular Disease

LDL cholesterol is not inherently dangerous. Oxidized LDL — LDL that has been attacked by reactive oxygen species — is dangerous. Oxidized LDL is preferentially taken up by macrophages in the arterial wall, forming foam cells, initiating the inflammatory cascade that produces atherosclerotic plaque. Vitamin C, vitamin E, selenium, and glutathione are the primary defenders of LDL against oxidative modification. Their insufficiency allows LDL oxidation to proceed, initiating the arterial disease that decades of lipid-lowering therapy has attempted to manage downstream.

Cancer Initiation

Oxidative damage to DNA — 8-hydroxydeoxyguanosine (8-OHdG) is the most studied marker — is among the most common mechanisms of cancer initiation. The body repairs oxidative DNA damage through a suite of enzymes that include glutathione-dependent steps and selenium-dependent thioredoxin reductase activity. When antioxidant defense is inadequate, oxidative DNA damage accumulates faster than repair mechanisms can address it. The Bruce Ames triage theory predicts that DNA repair is among the first processes sacrificed when micronutrients are insufficient — making chronic subclinical antioxidant insufficiency a plausible cancer risk factor that requires no single dramatic exposure.

Neurological Degeneration

The brain consumes approximately twenty percent of the body's oxygen despite comprising only two percent of its mass — making it among the most oxidatively stressed organs in the body. Neurons have high polyunsaturated fatty acid content in their membranes, making them particularly vulnerable to lipid peroxidation. Oxidative damage to mitochondria in neurons is now recognized as a central mechanism in Alzheimer's disease, Parkinson's disease, and ALS. The antioxidant defense in neuronal mitochondria — primarily MnSOD (manganese) and glutathione — is the first line of protection. Its insufficiency is an upstream contributor to neurodegenerative conditions that are being treated decades after the oxidative damage has accumulated.

Premature Aging

The free radical theory of aging — proposed by Denham Harman in 1956 — remains the most parsimonious explanation for why cells accumulate damage over time and eventually lose their functional integrity. Mitochondrial DNA is particularly vulnerable because it lacks the histone protection of nuclear DNA and is located adjacent to the primary source of reactive oxygen species generation. Mitochondrial DNA mutations accumulate with age; the rate of accumulation correlates with antioxidant defense status. Adequate antioxidant nutrition does not prevent aging, but inadequate antioxidant nutrition accelerates it through measurable and mechanistically understood pathways.

VI. The Web of Dependencies

The antioxidant orchestra is the most interdependent section of the entire nutritional symphony. The cascade of regeneration — vitamin E to vitamin C to glutathione to glutathione reductase (riboflavin + niacin) — means that every member of the network depends on every other member for its effectiveness. A person with adequate selenium but depleted glutathione has selenium sitting idle — the enzyme that contains it cannot complete its cycle. A person with high vitamin C intake but depleted glutathione cannot recycle the vitamin C. A person with adequate glutathione but depleted riboflavin and niacin cannot regenerate the oxidized glutathione. The network fails where any link fails.

The connections to other clusters deserve emphasis. The antioxidant network depends on the energy network (Cluster 1) for NADPH — the reducing currency that drives glutathione regeneration. It depends on the gut (Cluster 2) for the absorption of selenium, zinc, copper, and vitamin C. It depends on the methylation network (Cluster 9) for cysteine, one of glutathione's three amino acid components. And it depends on the amino acid network (Cluster 11) for glycine, another glutathione component that is chronically underconsumed in modern diets.

> *David's multivitamin provided the recommended daily amounts of vitamin C and E and selenium. What it did not provide was the full network those nutrients require to operate: adequate riboflavin and niacin to regenerate glutathione, adequate glycine and cysteine to build it, adequate manganese for MnSOD, adequate copper and zinc for Cu/Zn-SOD, and adequate alpha-lipoic acid to reset the entire system. A musician needs more than a score. They need an orchestra.*

VII. Questions Worth Asking

For a person experiencing slow wound healing, easy bruising, persistent fatigue despite adequate sleep and energy intake, recurrent infections, or a family history of early cardiovascular disease or neurodegenerative conditions — the antioxidant defense system represents an upstream territory that routine medicine does not explore.

Serum selenium and red blood cell selenium provide complementary pictures of selenium status. Plasma glutathione and erythrocyte glutathione measure the body's master antioxidant reserve. Plasma 8-OHdG is a validated marker of oxidative DNA damage. Serum alpha-tocopherol (vitamin E) is assessable but must be interpreted relative to total lipid content. Plasma ascorbate reflects recent vitamin C intake; whole blood ascorbate reflects longer-term status. Plasma copper and zinc alongside Cu/Zn-SOD activity provide a more functional picture of the SOD system than either mineral alone.

> *The information in this chapter is presented for educational purposes and does not constitute medical advice. Testing for antioxidant status and any interventions based on such testing should be discussed with a qualified healthcare professional. The author is not a clinician and does not offer clinical recommendations for any individual.*

VIII. David's Shield, Reconsidered

David's multivitamin contained the RDA for vitamin C, vitamin E, and selenium. It did not contain alpha-lipoic acid, glycine, N-acetylcysteine, riboflavin, or niacin in quantities that would support full glutathione regeneration. His diet was moderate in protein and low in organ meats — the richest dietary sources of both alpha-lipoic acid and the amino acids required for glutathione synthesis. His exercise, while health-promoting, was generating significant oxidative stress that his antioxidant network was not fully equipped to neutralize.

The slow wound healing, the easy bruising, the prolonged muscle soreness — these were not symptoms of any diagnosable disease. They were signals of a system under oxidative stress that was not being adequately defended. The fire was spreading further than it should before being contained, and accumulating the kind of damage — to lipids, to proteins, to DNA — that does not announce itself dramatically until it has accumulated for years.

David did not need a diagnosis. He needed a different question: not what is wrong, but whether the network that protects him from the combustion products of being alive is complete and functional. The tests that would answer that question were never ordered. The conversation that would raise it never happened.

For the Clinically Curious

The Glutathione Regeneration Cascade — Enzyme Biochemistry

Glutathione peroxidase (GPx) converts 2 GSH + H_2O_2 → GSSG + 2 H_2O, producing oxidized glutathione (GSSG). Glutathione reductase (GR) then reduces GSSG back to 2 GSH using NADPH as the electron donor: GSSG + NADPH + H^+ → 2 GSH + $NADP^+$. NADPH is generated primarily by glucose-6-phosphate dehydrogenase (G6PD) in the pentose phosphate pathway, using riboflavin (FAD) as cofactor and $NADP^+$ as substrate. G6PD deficiency — the most common enzymatic disorder in humans, affecting approximately 400 million people globally — therefore impairs glutathione regeneration under oxidative stress, explaining why G6PD-deficient individuals are at risk of hemolysis from oxidant exposures including certain drugs, fava beans, and infections. The NADPH connection means that niacin and riboflavin status directly determines the capacity for glutathione regeneration.

SOD Isoforms — Anatomical Distribution and Clinical Relevance

Three SOD isoforms exist in mammals: Cu/Zn-SOD (SOD1) in the cytoplasm; MnSOD (SOD2) in the mitochondrial matrix; and extracellular Cu/Zn-SOD (SOD3) in the extracellular space and plasma. SOD2 is mitochondrially encoded and upregulated in response to oxidative stress through NF-κB and AP-1 signaling. The Val16Ala variant (rs4880) in the SOD2 gene reduces mitochondrial targeting efficiency, producing a measurable reduction in mitochondrial MnSOD activity in heterozygous and homozygous carriers. Population frequency of the Ala allele is approximately 50% in European populations, making this one of the most common functional genetic variants in human biology and a compelling example of genetic variation that creates differential nutritional requirements (in this case, for manganese).

8-Hydroxydeoxyguanosine — Biomarker of Oxidative DNA Damage

8-OHdG is formed by the hydroxyl radical's attack on the C8 position of guanine in DNA. It is both a mutagenic lesion (causing G→T transversions when misread by DNA polymerase) and a validated biomarker of systemic oxidative stress. Urinary 8-OHdG reflects the steady-state balance between oxidative DNA damage generation and base excision repair (BER) — a balance that is directly sensitive to antioxidant nutrient status. Urinary 8-OHdG is elevated in cancer patients, in smokers, in diabetics, and in individuals with low plasma antioxidant concentrations. Intervention studies supplementing antioxidant networks — particularly combined vitamin C, vitamin E, and selenium — have shown significant reductions in urinary 8-OHdG, providing mechanistic evidence that nutritional antioxidant status directly affects genomic integrity.

NAC and Glycine as Glutathione Precursors — Clinical

Evidence

A randomized controlled trial (Kumar et al., Clinical Nutrition, 2021) demonstrated that elderly subjects (70–80 years) supplemented with N-acetylcysteine (1.33g/day) and glycine (1.67g/day) for 24 weeks restored red blood cell glutathione concentrations to levels comparable to young healthy adults, and significantly improved glutathione synthesis rates, oxidative stress markers (plasma 8-OHdG and F2-isoprostanes), mitochondrial fuel oxidation, body composition, muscle strength, exercise capacity, cognitive function, and insulin resistance compared to placebo. This is among the most comprehensive demonstrations available of the systemic consequences of glutathione insufficiency in aging and the clinical impact of glutathione precursor restoration.

Cluster 5

The Structural Architects

How Twelve Nutrients Build and Maintain the Physical Scaffolding of the Body — and Why Osteoporosis, Arterial Disease, and Connective Tissue Failure Are Nutritional Stories Medicine Has Mislabeled

> *"The body is not a machine that wears out. It is a structure that is continuously rebuilt — and like all structures, the quality of its rebuilding depends entirely on the quality of its materials."*

I. The Body That Rebuilds Itself

Elena is sixty-one years old. Her most recent bone density scan returned a T-score of -2.7, placing her in the osteoporosis range. Her physician prescribed a bisphosphonate — a drug that reduces bone resorption by inhibiting the osteoclasts that break down old bone. It is a rational, evidence-based intervention for improving bone density on subsequent DEXA scans.

What Elena was not told is that bone is not a mineral deposit. It is a living composite material — approximately thirty percent organic matrix, primarily collagen, and seventy percent mineral, primarily calcium phosphate crystals. The collagen matrix is built first. The mineral deposits within it second. A scaffold must exist before it can be loaded. Bisphosphonate therapy improves bone mineral density. It does not improve the collagen matrix in which that mineral is deposited. A bone with abundant mineral deposited in a deficient collagen matrix may show improved DEXA scores while remaining structurally fragile — more likely to fracture under real-world loading than the numbers suggest.

Nobody checked Elena's copper. Nobody assessed her vitamin C. Nobody asked about her lysyl oxidase — the copper-dependent enzyme that cross-links collagen fibers into the structural matrix that makes bone capable of bearing load rather than simply holding mineral. Nobody connected her borderline HDL — also a consequence of copper insufficiency — to the same upstream cause that was quietly degrading her skeletal architecture.

The structural architects of the human body — the nutrients that build, maintain, and repair its physical scaffolding — are among the most consequential and most neglected in clinical medicine. This chapter is about them.

II. Meet the Cast

Twelve musicians comprise the structural orchestra. Together, they manage the construction and continuous maintenance of bone, cartilage, tendon, ligament, arterial wall, skin, and every other collagen-rich tissue in the body.

- **Copper** — Cofactor for lysyl oxidase — the enzyme that cross-links collagen and elastin fibers into their mature, load-bearing form. Without copper, the scaffolding is assembled but not locked together.
- **Vitamin C** — Cofactor for prolyl hydroxylase and lysyl hydroxylase — the enzymes that modify proline and lysine in newly synthesized collagen chains, enabling them to fold into the collagen triple helix. Without vitamin C, collagen cannot be structurally completed.
- **Glycine** — The most abundant amino acid in collagen — comprising approximately thirty percent of its total amino acid content. Every third residue in the collagen triple helix is glycine. No glycine, no triple helix.
- **Proline** — The amino acid that forms the characteristic helical kinks in the collagen chain. Hydroxyproline — proline modified by prolyl hydroxylase (which requires vitamin C and iron) — is the most diagnostic amino acid in mature collagen.
- **Lysine** — Required for collagen cross-linking through hydroxylation (requiring vitamin C and iron) and subsequent modification by lysyl oxidase (requiring copper). Also the amino acid from which carnitine is synthesized.
- **Vitamin A** — Regulates the expression of collagen genes and the differentiation of fibroblasts — the cells that synthesize

collagen. Retinoic acid directly controls the transcription of collagen-encoding genes.

- **Zinc** — Required for the metalloproteinases that remodel collagen — the enzymes that break down old collagen to make way for new synthesis. Without adequate zinc, collagen remodeling is impaired.
- **Phosphorus** — The Bone Mineral Partner. Forms hydroxyapatite crystals with calcium, constituting the mineral phase of bone. Also the structural backbone of DNA, RNA, and every phospholipid membrane. Its balance with dietary calcium, regulated by vitamin D and PTH, determines bone mineralisation quality and arterial calcification risk.
- **Silicon** — Structural component of the proteoglycan ground substance that surrounds collagen fibers in cartilage and bone. Required for the cross-linking of collagen in bone matrix. Among the most overlooked structural minerals.
- **Vitamin K2** — Directs calcium into bone through the carboxylation of osteocalcin — the bone matrix protein that binds calcium. Without K2-dependent carboxylation, osteocalcin cannot bind calcium properly, and supplemental calcium may deposit in soft tissues rather than bone.
- **Manganese** — Required for glycosaminoglycan synthesis — the production of the ground substance molecules (chondroitin sulfate, keratan sulfate, hyaluronic acid) that form the cartilaginous matrix in joints and the interstitial matrix throughout connective tissue.
- **Boron** — Facilitates the bone-mineral system: improves calcium and magnesium retention, supports activation of

vitamin D, and modulates steroid hormone activity.

These twelve musicians together produce the material reality of the body's physical architecture. Their sufficiency determines whether the scaffold is robust or fragile, whether wounds heal or linger, whether arteries maintain their elasticity or stiffen, whether joints absorb load or degrade under it.

III. How Structural Tissue Is Built — A Map for the General Reader

The Collagen Story

Collagen is the most abundant protein in the human body, constituting approximately thirty percent of total protein content. It is the primary structural molecule of bone, tendon, ligament, cartilage, skin, blood vessel walls, and virtually every other connective tissue. There are at least twenty-eight distinct collagen types, but the structural logic is the same in all of them: three protein chains wound around each other in a right-handed triple helix, connected by cross-links that give the fiber its tensile strength.

The production of mature, functional collagen follows a precise sequence, and each step requires specific nutrients. First, fibroblasts transcribe and translate procollagen chains from genes that require vitamin A for their expression. The new chains are rich in proline and lysine, which are then modified by prolyl hydroxylase and lysyl hydroxylase — enzymes that require both iron and vitamin C as cofactors. Without these modifications, the three chains cannot fold into the triple helix. Without the triple helix, the molecule cannot leave the cell.

Once secreted outside the cell, the procollagen is cleaved to tropocollagen, which spontaneously assembles into fibrils. These fibrils are then locked into their final mature form by lysyl oxidase — the copper-dependent enzyme that creates covalent cross-links between adjacent tropocollagen molecules, dramatically increasing the tensile strength of the resulting fiber. This final cross-linking step is what makes collagen capable of bearing the mechanical loads that tendons, bone, and arterial walls experience continuously. Without copper, the fibrils form but remain unlocked, like a chain whose links are assembled but not welded.

Bone — More Than a Mineral

Bone is a two-component material: a collagen matrix that provides tensile strength and flexibility, and a mineral phase — primarily hydroxyapatite, a calcium phosphate crystal — that provides compressive strength and hardness. The two components work together to create a material that is simultaneously strong, flexible, and resistant to fracture under real-world loading conditions. Neither component alone produces bone with these properties. A bone with abundant mineral but deficient collagen matrix is brittle — it holds compressive load but fractures under bending. This is the structural reality behind the observation that bisphosphonate-treated bones can show improved DEXA scores while paradoxically increasing the risk of atypical femoral fractures in some patients.

Vitamin K2 governs where calcium deposits in the body. Osteocalcin — the major non-collagenous protein in bone matrix — binds calcium and holds it within the bone scaffold, but only when it has been carboxylated by a K2-dependent enzyme, gamma-carboxylase. Uncarboxylated osteocalcin cannot bind calcium. In vitamin K2 insufficiency, osteocalcin remains uncarboxylated, the mineral phase of bone is less effectively anchored to the matrix, and simultaneously, calcium that should be depositing in bone may instead deposit in arterial walls — contributing to vascular calcification. The arterial and skeletal consequences of vitamin K2 insufficiency are therefore two expressions of the same upstream biochemical failure.

IV. The Musicians, One by One

Copper — The Cross-Linker

Lysyl oxidase requires copper as its catalytic cofactor. The enzyme oxidizes specific lysine and hydroxylysine residues in collagen and elastin chains to aldehydes, which then condense spontaneously to form covalent cross-links between adjacent molecules. These cross-links are the structural bonds that give mature collagen its extraordinary tensile strength — tendons can withstand forces several times body weight because of lysyl oxidase-mediated cross-linking — and that give elastin in arterial walls their capacity to expand and recoil with each heartbeat without fatiguing.

Copper deficiency produces structural consequences that mirror the histology of the cross-linking failure: tendons that rupture under normal loading, arterial walls that dilate and bulge rather than maintaining pressure, skin that heals poorly and tears easily, and bones whose collagen matrix is inadequate to hold the mineral content that DEXA would record. Menkes disease — the genetic condition of copper malabsorption — produces all of these consequences in the most dramatic possible form, including kinking of hair (called kinky hair disease) that reflects the abnormal structure of keratin, a protein that also requires lysyl oxidase-mediated cross-linking.

Its essential partners: *Copper and iron work together in collagen maturation. Iron is required for prolyl and lysyl hydroxylase — the enzymes that modify the collagen chains before they leave the cell. Copper is required for lysyl oxidase — the enzyme that cross-links them after secretion. Both must be adequate for the full collagen production sequence to complete. Vitamin C is required by both iron-containing enzyme steps.*

Vitamin C — The Scaffolding Completer

Prolyl hydroxylase and lysyl hydroxylase — the enzymes that modify collagen chains — require ferrous iron at their active sites and ascorbate (vitamin C) as an electron donor to maintain that iron in its reduced, active form. Vitamin C is consumed stoichiometrically in this reaction — each modification event consumes one molecule of ascorbate. In vitamin C deficiency, prolyl and lysyl hydroxylation is impaired. The resulting collagen chains cannot fold into the triple helix. They are degraded within the cell, or secreted in incompletely processed form and incorporated into defective matrix.

This is the molecular basis of scurvy: the bleeding gums, the reopening of old wounds, the perifollicular hemorrhages, and the fatal internal bleeding represent the systematic failure of collagen throughout the body when vitamin C is absent. The modern equivalent is not scurvy but the subclinical insufficiency that produces bleeding gums, slow wound healing, impaired arterial wall collagen, and reduced bone matrix quality in populations whose vitamin C intake prevents overt deficiency while falling short of the amounts required for optimal collagen synthesis.

Margaret's bleeding gums were a signal. They were the most accessible and most visible manifestation of a systemic connective tissue insufficiency that was also affecting her arterial walls, her immune cell function, and the structural integrity of every collagen-rich tissue in her body. Her dentist recommended flossing. Nobody recommended ascorbate assessment.

Its essential partner: *Vitamin C is regenerated by glutathione after its role in collagen synthesis. This connects the structural network to the antioxidant network: adequate glutathione preserves vitamin C availability for collagen synthesis. In glutathione-depleted states, vitamin C is irreversibly consumed* *and collagen synthesis slows even when dietary vitamin C intake is adequate.*

Glycine — The Collagen Backbone

Glycine is the smallest amino acid — a single hydrogen atom where other amino acids have larger side chains. This smallness is not incidental. The collagen triple helix requires a glycine at every third position because only glycine is small enough to fit in the central space of the helix. If any other amino acid substitutes for glycine, the helix cannot form at that position, and the resulting structural defect produces localized weakness.

Glycine is classified as a non-essential amino acid — meaning the body can synthesize it — but the synthesis is insufficient to meet demand under most conditions. Research has estimated that the body can synthesize approximately three grams of glycine per day, while optimal collagen synthesis may require ten to fifteen grams per day for an adult. The gap between synthesis capacity and requirement is filled by dietary intake. Modern low-protein diets, and particularly diets low in collagen-rich foods — bone broth, skin, cartilage, organ meats — may be systematically insufficient in glycine. A 2019 paper estimated that glycine deficiency may be the most prevalent nutritional insufficiency in Western populations that has not yet been formally recognized as a clinical problem.

Its essential partners: *Glycine works in precise stoichiometry with proline and lysine in the collagen chain. It is also one of the three amino acids required for glutathione synthesis — connecting* *the structural and antioxidant networks at the amino acid level. The body cannot maximally support both collagen synthesis and glutathione production if glycine is insufficient; it must triage.*

Vitamin K2 — The Calcium Director

Vitamin K2 — distinct from vitamin K1, which is involved in blood clotting — activates matrix Gla proteins (MGP) and osteocalcin through gamma-carboxylation, a modification that allows these proteins to bind calcium ions. MGP is the primary inhibitor of soft tissue calcification: it is produced by vascular smooth muscle cells and cartilage, and in its active (carboxylated) form, it prevents calcium from depositing in arterial walls and joints. In its inactive (uncarboxylated) form — the state produced by K2 insufficiency — MGP cannot perform this function.

Population studies consistently find that low dietary vitamin K2 intake is associated with higher coronary artery calcification scores and higher cardiovascular mortality. The Rotterdam Study — one of the largest epidemiological assessments of K2 — found that high menaquinone (K2) intake was associated with a fifty-seven percent reduction in cardiovascular mortality compared to low intake. The mechanism is the activation of MGP in arterial walls: adequate K2 keeps arteries soft by preventing calcium deposition; insufficient K2 allows the arterial calcification that stiffens vessels and raises cardiovascular risk.

The practical implication extends to calcium supplementation. A person taking calcium supplements without adequate vitamin K2 is providing additional mineral substrate for deposition in soft tissues as well as bone. The K2-calcium combination — with the routing function K2 provides — is a more physiologically coherent approach than calcium alone.

Its essential partners: *Vitamin K2 works with vitamin D, which drives calcium absorption from the gut and increases circulating calcium levels. Without K2 to route that calcium appropriately, increased vitamin D-driven calcium absorption may increase soft tissue calcification risk alongside bone mineralisation. The D-K2 pair should be understood together. Magnesium is required for vitamin D activation and also for the bone crystal structure into which the directed calcium is ultimately deposited.*

Boron — The Bone-Mineral Facilitator

Boron is the quiet partner in the bone-mineral system. It does not build the scaffold directly, as copper and vitamin C do, nor form the mineral itself, as phosphorus does. It governs how efficiently the other minerals are kept and used. Boron reduces the urinary loss of both calcium and magnesium, and it supports the step that converts vitamin D into its active hormonal form — meaning a boron insufficiency can blunt the effect of otherwise adequate calcium, magnesium, and vitamin D at the same time. It also influences the activity of the steroid hormones, including the estrogen and testosterone that govern bone maintenance across a lifespan (a role taken up in Cluster 6).

Boron is among the least measured of the minerals that matter to structural tissue. It appears on no standard panel, and its dietary sources — chiefly fruit, nuts, and legumes — are among the foods most reduced in processed dietary patterns. The question worth asking is not whether a boron level is "low" against a reference range that barely exists, but whether a diet stripped of its plant sources has quietly removed one of the facilitators that determines whether the rest of the bone-mineral system can do its work.

V. Phosphorus — The Architecture of Bone and Every Membrane

Phosphorus is the second most abundant mineral in the human body, present predominantly as phosphate (PO43-). In bone, phosphate combines with calcium to form hydroxyapatite — Ca10(PO4)6(OH)2 — the crystal that constitutes approximately seventy percent of bone's dry weight and provides its compressive strength and hardness. Without adequate phosphorus, the mineral phase of bone cannot be properly crystallised regardless of calcium or vitamin D status. Hypophosphatemia produces osteomalacia — soft, incompletely mineralised bone that bends and fractures under normal loading. This is the phosphorus-deficiency bone disease, the direct counterpart of the calcium-deficiency disease rickets, and it is almost never mentioned in clinical discussions of osteoporosis despite phosphorus being an equal partner in the hydroxyapatite crystal that DEXA scans measure.

Beyond bone, phosphorus as phosphate is the structural backbone of DNA and RNA — the phosphodiester bonds linking nucleotides are phosphate bonds. Every cell division, every protein synthesis event, every gene expression change depends on phosphate. ATP — adenosine triphosphate, the energy currency of Cluster 1 — is three phosphate groups in series whose sequential hydrolysis releases the energy that every cellular process consumes. And phospholipids, the structural molecules of every cell membrane, are phosphate-containing lipids: remove the phosphate head group and the amphipathic character of the lipid bilayer dissolves. Phosphorus is not a supporting mineral. It is the molecular scaffold on which the chemistry of life is built.

The modern concern with phosphorus is not deficiency but dysregulation. Phosphate salts added as preservatives, leavening agents, and texture modifiers are the largest source of phosphorus in Western diets — and unlike the organic phosphorus in natural foods (which is absorbed at approximately sixty percent), inorganic phosphate additives are absorbed at nearly one hundred percent. Excessive phosphate elevates FGF-23, suppresses vitamin D activation, and disrupts the calcium-phosphorus ratio that governs hydroxyapatite crystal quality. High dietary phosphate from processed food is independently associated with cardiovascular mortality and accelerated kidney function decline — consequences of a mineral manipulation that entered the food supply as a technical convenience and whose population-level health effects were never systematically evaluated.

Its essential partners: *Calcium and phosphorus are regulated together by vitamin D and PTH — the ratio between them matters as much as their absolute levels. The optimal dietary calcium-to-phosphorus ratio is approximately 1:1; Western diets provide 1:2 to 1:3, with excess phosphate from food additives potentially impairing bone crystal quality. Magnesium occupies specific sites in the hydroxyapatite lattice, and adequate magnesium produces crystals of appropriate size and solubility for healthy bone remodeling. Vitamin K2 then directs calcium into the matrix through osteocalcin carboxylation — completing the four-mineral system that structural bone mineralisation requires.*

VI. The Modern Structural Crisis

The structural insufficiencies described in this chapter are not rare or exotic. They are built into the modern lifestyle through specific, identifiable mechanisms.

The Glycine Deficit

Traditional diets consumed the whole animal — including skin, joints, bone broth, cartilage, and organ meats that are rich in glycine and proline. Modern Western diets are dominated by skeletal muscle meat — chicken breast and other lean muscle meats — which is rich in methionine but relatively poor in glycine. The shift from whole-animal to muscle-meat consumption over the past century has produced a systematic reduction in dietary glycine that has been largely unrecognized because glycine's deficiency does not produce the kind of acute clinical syndrome that historically triggered recognition.

The Copper Depletion

The widespread use of high-dose zinc supplements — for immune support, testosterone, or skin health — reliably depletes copper through competitive inhibition of intestinal absorption. Copper's primary dietary sources — organ meats, shellfish, dark chocolate — are consumed infrequently in most Western diets. The combination produces the silent copper insufficiency that impairs lysyl oxidase, impairs collagen cross-linking, impairs Complex IV energy production, impairs superoxide dismutase antioxidant defense, and impairs iron mobilization — all while serum copper appears normal because ceruloplasmin rises with any inflammatory signal.

The Vitamin K2 Disappearance

Vitamin K2 is found primarily in fermented foods — natto (a Japanese fermented soybean product), certain aged cheeses, and fermented dairy products — and in organ meats and grass-fed animal products. As fermented foods have declined in the Western diet and as the proportion of meat from grain-fed rather than grass-fed animals has increased, dietary K2 intake has fallen dramatically. Population studies confirm that dietary menaquinone intake in Western countries is a fraction of that in Asian populations with higher natto consumption, and that this difference is reflected in measurably different rates of cardiovascular calcification and osteoporotic fracture.

VII. The Web of Dependencies

The structural network's interdependencies are among the most clinically important in this book, because they explain why the standard medical interventions for structural conditions so frequently produce partial results.

Calcium supplementation for osteoporosis without vitamin K2 may partly deposit calcium in arteries rather than bone. Calcium with K2 but without vitamin D fails because calcium is not absorbed. Vitamin D without magnesium fails because the enzyme that activates vitamin D requires magnesium. Collagen supplementation without vitamin C, glycine, and proline provides substrate for a synthesis process that lacks its enzymatic requirements. Bisphosphonate therapy that reduces bone resorption without improving the collagen matrix — which requires copper, vitamin C, glycine, and proline — improves the mineral quantity of bone without improving its structural quality.

The structural musicians must play together. The interventions that work in isolation — because a clinical trial tested one variable in a population whose other nutritional variables were uncontrolled — dramatically understate what the complete orchestra can produce when all musicians are present.

> *Elena's bisphosphonate will reduce her bone resorption and improve her DEXA score. It will not improve the lysyl oxidase-mediated collagen cross-linking that determines whether her bone matrix can bear load. That requires copper. It will not improve the prolyl hydroxylase function that determines whether her collagen chains are structurally complete. That requires vitamin C and iron. It will not direct calcium into the bone matrix rather than her arterial walls. That requires vitamin K2. The drug addresses one variable in a multi-variable system. The system continues to fail at every other variable.*

VIII. Questions Worth Asking

For a person with osteoporosis, frequent fractures, slow wound healing, easy bruising, skin that heals poorly, joint pain, or documented arterial calcification — the structural network represents upstream territory that standard clinical management rarely assesses.

Serum copper and ceruloplasmin together (not serum copper alone) provide a picture of copper status. RBC copper is more accurate for longer-term status. Plasma vitamin C measures recent intake. Serum zinc alongside copper provides the ratio that is clinically more meaningful than either alone. Undercarboxylated osteocalcin in serum is the most direct measure of vitamin K2 activity in bone — higher values indicate K2 insufficiency. 25(OH)D for vitamin D status alongside PTH provides the regulatory context. Serum and urine collagen crosslinks (pyridinoline, deoxypyridinoline) assess collagen remodeling rates.

The information in this chapter is educational and does not constitute clinical advice. The management of osteoporosis, cardiovascular disease, and connective tissue conditions requires individualized clinical assessment and should be discussed with qualified healthcare professionals. The author does not offer clinical recommendations for any individual, and the nutritional factors described here are presented to inform rather than to guide specific therapeutic decisions.

IX. Elena's Architecture, Reconsidered

Elena's DEXA scan showed low bone mineral density. It showed nothing about the collagen matrix in which that mineral resides. Her copper had never been measured. Her vitamin C status had never been assessed. Her vitamin K2 intake — from a diet low in fermented foods and grass-fed animal products — had never been discussed. Her zinc supplement, which she had been taking for two years for immune support, had been silently competing with copper for intestinal absorption throughout that period.

The bisphosphonate prescribed to her is a rational response to the number on the DEXA scan. It is an incomplete response to the biology underlying that number. The skeleton Elena needed was one whose collagen matrix was as well-supported as its mineral content — an outcome that the bisphosphonate cannot achieve and that the nutritional network described in this chapter could help provide if it were assessed and addressed.

What Elena deserved was not just a bone density scan and a prescription. She deserved an investigation that asked why her collagen matrix was insufficient and what the full complement of structural nutrients — copper, vitamin C, glycine, vitamin K2, manganese, silicon — was doing in her body. Those tests were not ordered. That conversation was not available. The architecture was failing at its foundation while the interventions addressed only its mineral surface.

For the Clinically Curious

Lysyl Oxidase — Biochemistry and Clinical Manifestations of Deficiency

Lysyl oxidase (LOX) is a copper-dependent amine oxidase that oxidizes the epsilon-amino groups of lysine and hydroxylysine residues in collagen and elastin chains to reactive aldehydes. These aldehydes then undergo condensation reactions — primarily aldol condensation and Schiff base formation — to form the covalent intermolecular cross-links that stabilize fibrillar collagen and elastin networks. The specific cross-links formed depend on tissue type: bone collagen is characterized by pyridinoline and deoxypyridinoline cross-links; arterial elastin by desmosine cross-links. LOX deficiency — whether from copper insufficiency or from the rare mutations causing occipital horn syndrome (a mild allelic variant of Menkes disease) — produces a characteristic connective tissue phenotype: aortic aneurysm (from impaired elastin cross-linking), skeletal abnormalities, joint hypermobility, and skin fragility. The LOX-copper dependency means that any condition producing copper insufficiency — whether from dietary inadequacy, excessive zinc intake, malabsorption, or gastric bypass surgery — can produce subclinical connective tissue fragility through the same mechanism.

Undercarboxylated Osteocalcin — Clinical Assessment of Vitamin K2 Status

Osteocalcin is synthesized by osteoblasts and represents the primary non-collagenous protein in bone matrix. It contains three glutamate residues that are gamma-carboxylated by the K2-dependent enzyme gamma-glutamyl carboxylase (GGCX) to produce gamma-carboxyglutamate (Gla) residues, which can chelate calcium ions. Undercarboxylated osteocalcin (ucOC) — the fraction lacking Gla residues — cannot effectively bind calcium and circulates in blood as a measure of K2 insufficiency. The %ucOC (percentage of total osteocalcin that is undercarboxylated) is a more sensitive indicator of K2 status than serum K2 concentrations, which are poorly standardized. Studies consistently find %ucOC above fifty percent in Western populations not consuming fermented K2-rich foods or supplements, suggesting widespread K2 insufficiency by functional criteria.

Silicon — The Overlooked Structural Mineral

Silicon (as orthosilicic acid, $Si(OH)4$) is the bioavailable form in which silicon influences collagen synthesis and mineralisation. Silicon is concentrated at the mineralisation front of bone — the site of active hydroxyapatite crystal nucleation — and is required for the hydroxylation of proline in collagen synthesis through an incompletely characterized mechanism. The most cited evidence comes from epidemiological studies showing positive correlations between dietary silicon intake (from whole grains, root vegetables, and beer) and bone mineral density in pre-menopausal women. Orthosilicic acid supplementation has shown modest bone-supportive effects in several clinical trials. Silicon is present in refining process residues — meaning that food processing reduces silicon content. The RDA for silicon has not been established, though estimated adequate intakes have been proposed in the range of 20-50mg/day (Jugdaohsingh et al., American Journal of Clinical Nutrition, 2002).

Glycine Deficiency — The Underrecognized Structural Insufficiency

De novo glycine synthesis from serine via serine hydroxymethyltransferase (SHMT) produces approximately 3g/day in an adult. Estimated requirement for glycine balance — accounting for collagen synthesis, glutathione production, creatine synthesis, bile acid conjugation, and N-methylation — ranges from 10 to 15g/day, suggesting a functional deficit of 7-12g/day in individuals not consuming collagen-rich foods. Urinary hydroxyproline and hydroxylysine are indirect markers of collagen turnover, and low values in the context of osteoporosis or poor wound healing may indicate inadequate collagen synthesis substrate alongside other structural nutrients. Supplemental glycine at doses of 3-10g/day is well-tolerated and has shown clinical benefits in sleep quality, metabolic syndrome, and inflammatory bowel disease in randomized trials, consistent with its systemic structural and anti-inflammatory roles.

Cluster 6

The Hormonal Regulators

How Twelve Nutrients Govern the Body's Command and Control System — and Why Treating Thyroid, Adrenal, and Metabolic Conditions Without Addressing Their Nutritional Root Is Medicine Treating a Broken Speedometer

> *"The hormone is the messenger. The nutrients are what make the messenger, deliver it, and allow the receiving cell to read it. Treat only the messenger, and the message system remains broken."*

I. The Command System That Runs on Minerals

James is forty-four years old. He has been on levothyroxine for six years for Hashimoto's thyroiditis. His TSH is well-controlled. He continues to feel cold when others are comfortable. His hair is thinning. His energy is unreliable. His weight is stubbornly elevated despite a calorie-controlled diet. He has been told his thyroid medication is working — his TSH is in range — and that his remaining symptoms are likely stress or age.

What James has not been told is that the thyroid gland requires five nutrients to synthesize thyroid hormones. That the conversion of the inactive T4 — which is what levothyroxine provides — to the active T3 that his cells can use requires a sixth. That the receptor in his cells through which T3 signals requires a seventh. That his thyroid gland is being progressively destroyed by autoimmune antibodies whose production is influenced by an eighth. And that the iodine required for the hormones themselves, and the amino acid tyrosine from which their backbone is constructed, complete the essential complement.

His TSH is normal because his medication is replacing the hormone. The system that should have produced that hormone naturally — from thyroid gland synthesis through liver conversion to cellular receptor signaling — is impaired at multiple points that no blood panel in six years of treatment has been assessed.

II. Meet the Cast

Twelve musicians comprise the hormonal regulatory orchestra described in this chapter. They govern the thyroid, adrenal, pancreatic, and sex hormone systems — the body's primary command and control infrastructure.

- **Iodine** — The mineral component of thyroid hormones T3 and T4. Without iodine, thyroid hormones literally cannot be constructed — they are iodinated tyrosine residues.
- **Tyrosine** — The amino acid backbone of thyroid hormones — T3 is triiodothyronine (three iodine atoms on one tyrosine), T4 is tetraiodothyronine (four iodines on one tyrosine). Without tyrosine, iodine has nothing to attach to.
- **Selenium** — The mineral required by deiodinase enzymes — the enzymes that remove one iodine atom from T4 to produce the active T3. Without selenium, T4 cannot be converted to T3 regardless of how much thyroid hormone is synthesized.
- **Iron** — Required by thyroid peroxidase — the enzyme that iodates tyrosine residues in the thyroid gland to produce thyroid hormones. Iron deficiency impairs thyroid hormone synthesis directly.
- **Zinc** — Required for thyroid hormone receptor function — the cellular protein through which T3 produces its biological effects. Without adequate zinc, T3 cannot signal effectively even when its concentrations are normal.
- **Vitamin A** — Regulates thyroid hormone receptor expression and function. Retinoic acid forms dimers with the thyroid hormone receptor at nuclear binding sites, modulating the receptor's sensitivity to T3.
- **Potassium** — The Electrical Conductor. The primary intracellular cation, maintaining the electrochemical gradient that enables nerve conduction, cardiac rhythm, vascular smooth muscle relaxation, and blood pressure

regulation. Regulated by aldosterone and insulin — both hormonal players in this cluster.

- **Chromium** — Potentiates insulin signaling at the receptor level, enhancing glucose uptake in response to insulin. Deficiency contributes to insulin resistance independent of body weight or dietary composition.
- **Vanadium** — Mimics insulin at the receptor, supporting glucose uptake; a trace partner to chromium in maintaining insulin sensitivity.
- **Magnesium** — Required for insulin receptor phosphorylation — the molecular event that initiates insulin signaling inside the cell. Also required for the ATP-dependent glucose transporters that move glucose into cells.
- **Vitamin C** — Concentrated in higher amounts in the adrenal glands than in any other tissue, where it is consumed in the synthesis of cortisol and adrenaline. Chronic stress depletes adrenal vitamin C continuously.
- **Vitamin D** — Functions as a steroid hormone, activating gene expression through nuclear receptors in virtually every cell type. Its receptors are present in thyroid tissue, pancreatic beta cells, immune cells, and neurons — connecting it to every hormonal system in the book.

III. The Thyroid Symphony — Most Carefully Played

The thyroid axis is among the most complex hormonal systems in human biology, and it is the one in which nutritional insufficiency most commonly produces clinical consequences that are pharmacologically managed without nutritional investigation.

Synthesis — Five Nutrients for Two Hormones

Thyroid hormone synthesis begins in the follicular cells of the thyroid gland with the production of thyroglobulin — a large glycoprotein scaffold to which iodine is then attached at specific tyrosine residues by thyroid peroxidase. This enzyme is iron-dependent: iron deficiency impairs thyroid peroxidase activity and reduces thyroid hormone synthesis even when iodine intake is adequate. The iodine that is attached to thyroglobulin must come from dietary intake — the body cannot synthesize it. Tyrosine, the amino acid backbone, must also be provided by diet or synthesized from phenylalanine — a process that can be rate-limiting under conditions of low protein intake.

When thyroid hormones are released from thyroglobulin into the circulation, the primary product is T4 — tetraiodothyronine — which is largely inactive at the cellular level. T4 is a prohormone — a storage and transport form that must be converted to T3 to exert biological effects. This conversion is performed by deiodinase enzymes, primarily in the liver, kidney, and target tissues.

Deiodinase enzymes are selenoproteins — they require selenium at their active sites, in the form of selenocysteine, to perform the deiodination reaction. This is the step that explains why James continues to feel hypothyroid on adequate levothyroxine with a normal TSH: his T4 is being replaced, but his selenium status — never measured — may be insufficient for efficient T4-to-T3 conversion.

Signaling — Where Zinc and Vitamin A Operate

At the cellular level, T3 enters the nucleus and binds to the thyroid hormone receptor (THR) — a zinc finger transcription factor. The zinc finger structure of the receptor is essential for its ability to bind DNA at thyroid hormone response elements and activate or suppress gene expression. Zinc insufficiency impairs zinc finger function in the thyroid hormone receptor, reducing the receptor's capacity to transduce T3 signals into biological effects. A patient with low-normal zinc and adequate T3 may have impaired thyroid hormone signaling at the receptor level — a deficit invisible to any standard thyroid function test.

Vitamin A (retinoic acid) forms heterodimeric complexes with the thyroid hormone receptor through retinoid X receptor (RXR) binding. The T3/THR complex and the retinoic acid/RXR complex bind to adjacent response elements in the DNA as a heterodimer, and the vitamin A component modulates the sensitivity of the receptor complex to T3. Vitamin A deficiency therefore impairs thyroid hormone signaling not by reducing T3 concentrations but by reducing the receptor system's ability to translate those concentrations into appropriate gene expression changes.

Autoimmunity — Where Selenium Acts Again

Hashimoto's thyroiditis — James's diagnosis — is an autoimmune condition in which antibodies against thyroid peroxidase (anti-TPO) and thyroglobulin (anti-TG) are produced by the immune system and gradually destroy thyroid tissue. Multiple randomized controlled trials have demonstrated that selenium supplementation significantly reduces anti-TPO and anti-TG antibody titres in Hashimoto's patients — by approximately thirty to forty percent in most studies — and improves the echogenicity of the thyroid on ultrasound, consistent with reduced inflammatory infiltration. The mechanism involves selenoprotein-mediated reduction of hydrogen peroxide in thyroid follicular cells: thyroid hormone synthesis generates hydrogen peroxide as a byproduct, and selenoprotein P and glutathione peroxidase neutralize it. In selenium deficiency, hydrogen peroxide accumulates in thyroid tissue, oxidizing thyroid proteins and generating neoepitopes that the immune system may recognize as foreign.

James's selenium was never measured. His anti-TPO antibodies were monitored annually as a marker of disease activity. The nutrient that randomized controlled trials have shown can reduce those antibodies by a third was never incorporated into his management. This is not a failure of the evidence — it is a failure of the framework.

IV. Potassium — The Body's Electrical Conductor

Potassium is the most abundant intracellular cation in the human body — ninety-eight percent of the body's potassium resides inside cells, maintaining the electrical charge difference across membranes that makes every excitable tissue function. Neurons fire, muscle contracts, and the heart beats rhythmically because of the electrochemical gradient sustained by the sodium-potassium ATPase pump, which moves three sodium ions out and two potassium ions in for every ATP molecule consumed. This pump accounts for twenty to forty percent of the body's total resting energy expenditure. Potassium is not a passenger in this process — it is the gradient the pump is building, and the gradient the entire nervous and cardiovascular system depends on to operate.

The hormonal connections are direct and clinically underappreciated. Aldosterone — the adrenal hormone that regulates sodium and potassium balance — is secreted in response to low blood potassium and drives potassium conservation by the kidney. Insulin stimulates cellular potassium uptake alongside glucose, coupling insulin resistance and potassium dysregulation biochemically. Cortisol, produced under chronic stress, promotes urinary potassium loss — connecting the adrenal stress response to potassium depletion through a mechanism that is invisible on standard blood panels. Margaret's decade of chronic stress, mediated through elevated cortisol, has been quietly increasing her urinary potassium losses alongside her magnesium losses. Her serum potassium has always been in range. Nobody connected it to her hypertension as an upstream contributor.

Potassium's role in blood pressure is among the most robustly documented nutrient-cardiovascular relationships in epidemiology. The INTERSALT study found that dietary potassium was as strongly inversely associated with blood pressure as dietary sodium was positively associated — yet clinical management of hypertension focuses almost exclusively on sodium restriction and pharmaceuticals, while the potassium side of the equation receives little systematic attention. Potassium directly relaxes vascular smooth muscle through hyperpolarisation of the membrane, reduces renal sodium reabsorption, and modulates the renin-angiotensin-aldosterone axis. A patient prescribed an ACE inhibitor or angiotensin receptor blocker for hypertension is being given a drug that partially mimics the downstream effects of adequate dietary potassium — without any assessment of whether that dietary potassium is adequate.

Its essential partners: *Potassium and magnesium are regulated together — magnesium deficiency impairs renal potassium conservation, making potassium depletion refractory to replacement unless magnesium is corrected simultaneously. This co-depletion is especially common with diuretic therapy and chronic stress. The sodium-potassium ATPase that maintains potassium gradients requires magnesium as a cofactor — magnesium-depleted cells lose potassium regardless of dietary intake.*

V. The Insulin-Glucose System

Chromium — The Insulin Sensitizer

Chromium — specifically chromium (III) — forms part of a low-molecular-weight complex called chromodulin (formerly called glucose tolerance factor) that potentiates insulin's action at the receptor level. When insulin binds to its receptor on the cell surface, chromodulin binds to the intracellular domain of the activated receptor and amplifies the downstream phosphorylation cascade that drives glucose uptake. Without adequate chromium, the insulin signal is transmitted less efficiently, and more insulin is required to achieve the same glucose uptake — a functional form of insulin resistance.

The clinical significance of chromium insufficiency is that it contributes to insulin resistance and impaired glucose tolerance in a population already experiencing epidemic metabolic dysfunction. Chromium is depleted by high-sugar diets — a cruel irony in which the dietary pattern most likely to produce insulin resistance also depletes the trace mineral most needed to maintain insulin sensitivity. Chromium is excreted in the urine in proportion to refined sugar consumption: each gram of sugar increases urinary chromium loss.

Vanadium — The Insulin Mimic

Where chromium amplifies insulin's signal, vanadium imitates it. In its dietary forms, vanadium inhibits the protein tyrosine phosphatases that switch the insulin receptor off; with those brakes eased, the receptor's glucose-uptake cascade runs longer on the same amount of insulin. The effect is insulin-like at the cellular level, which is why vanadium has been studied for its capacity to improve glucose tolerance and lower fasting glucose in insulin-resistant states.

The clinical picture mirrors chromium's: a trace mineral required in minute amounts, poorly represented on standard testing, and drawn from whole-food sources — mushrooms, shellfish, whole grains, and legumes — that a refined diet supplies less of. It is not a mineral to self-administer; higher supplemental doses carry their own safety questions and belong in a physician's hands. But as one of the two trace minerals that quietly condition how well insulin works, vanadium is part of the answer to why insulin resistance can develop and persist even after the more familiar levers have been pulled. The question worth asking is whether the trace-mineral foundation of glucose control is intact before concluding that the system itself has failed.

Magnesium — The Insulin Receptor Activator

The insulin receptor is a tyrosine kinase — it signals by phosphorylating tyrosine residues on downstream proteins. This phosphorylation requires ATP, and ATP requires magnesium for its biological activity. Magnesium deficiency therefore impairs insulin signaling at the most fundamental mechanistic level: the energy currency that drives the receptor cannot be activated without magnesium. Population studies consistently find that magnesium intake is inversely associated with type 2 diabetes risk, and that hypomagnesemia is significantly more prevalent in diabetic populations than in normoglycemic controls. The relationship is bidirectional: insulin resistance increases urinary magnesium loss, and magnesium deficiency worsens insulin resistance — a feedback loop that standard diabetes management does not typically address.

VI. The Adrenal System — Vitamin C's Primary Consumer

The adrenal glands are among the most metabolically demanding organs in the body during periods of stress. They synthesize cortisol, adrenaline, noradrenaline, DHEA, and aldosterone — a spectrum of hormones governing stress response, blood pressure, energy mobilization, immune modulation, and electrolyte balance. This synthesis requires substantial nutritional support.

The adrenal glands contain the highest concentration of vitamin C of any tissue in the body. Vitamin C is consumed in the synthesis of cortisol (the enzyme dopamine beta-hydroxylase, which produces noradrenaline from dopamine, is vitamin C dependent) and is depleted by ACTH stimulation and by the oxidative stress of acute stress responses. A person under chronic psychological stress is consuming adrenal vitamin C continuously — and the same stress that drives this consumption also increases cortisol, which increases magnesium excretion, which impairs energy metabolism, which reduces the capacity for the cellular repair that requires glutathione — which requires the vitamin C that the adrenals have consumed.

The nutritional cost of chronic stress is not metaphorical. It is biochemically specific: thiamine demand rises with metabolic rate, magnesium is excreted in proportion to cortisol, vitamin C is consumed by adrenal hormone synthesis, and B vitamins are consumed by the accelerated energy metabolism that stress demands. The fatigued person under chronic stress is nutritionally depleted in a highly specific and predictable pattern that could be measured and addressed. It is neither measured nor addressed.

VII. The Web of Dependencies

The hormonal network's interdependencies form some of the most clinically important patterns in this book:

Iodine requires selenium: T4 synthesis requires iodine; T4 activation requires selenium. Treating iodine deficiency or supplementing T4 without adequate selenium leaves the conversion step impaired. High iodine intake without adequate selenium increases hydrogen peroxide in the thyroid, potentially worsening Hashimoto's autoimmunity.

Selenium requires vitamin E: Glutathione peroxidase (selenium-dependent) protects the thyroid from hydrogen peroxide. Vitamin E protects selenoproteins from oxidative inactivation. Selenium and vitamin E are synergistic in thyroid protection.

Thyroid requires iron: Iron deficiency impairs thyroid peroxidase and reduces thyroid hormone synthesis. In populations with combined iron and iodine deficiency — common in developing countries — correcting iodine alone without iron produces inadequate thyroid hormone response.

Magnesium enables everything: Magnesium activates ATP, which drives insulin receptor phosphorylation, which enables glucose uptake, which provides the energy substrate that every hormonal synthesis reaction requires. Magnesium deficiency therefore impairs hormonal function at the most fundamental energetic level, across all glands simultaneously.

Vitamin D connects to all: Vitamin D receptors are present in thyroid tissue (modulating autoimmune risk), in pancreatic beta cells (modulating insulin secretion), in adrenal tissue, and in the immune cells whose activation determines the autoimmune risk in Hashimoto's. Vitamin D is the hormonal network's cross-system modulator.

> *James's thyroid medication replaced the hormone. It did not address the selenium insufficiency that impairs T4-to-T3 conversion. It did not address the zinc insufficiency that impairs thyroid receptor function. It did not address the iron insufficiency that impairs thyroid peroxidase activity. It did not address the selenium insufficiency that allows anti-TPO antibodies to continue destroying his gland. The TSH is normal. The system behind it remains broken at five separate points. The medication has quietened the alarm. The fire has not been extinguished.*

VIII. Questions Worth Asking

For a person with hypothyroidism who continues to feel hypothyroid on adequate levothyroxine — one of the most common clinical frustrations in endocrinology — the nutritional assessment described in this cluster represents a legitimate, evidence-grounded upstream investigation.

Serum selenium and RBC selenium provide complementary pictures of selenium status — including whether selenium is available for the deiodinase enzymes that convert T4 to T3. Free T3 alongside free T4 reveals the efficiency of T4-to-T3 conversion. Anti-TPO and anti-TG antibody titres assessed in the context of selenium status give a picture of whether selenium intervention might reduce the autoimmune burden. Serum and RBC zinc alongside thyroid function provides the receptor function context. RBC magnesium alongside fasting insulin and HOMA-IR provides the insulin resistance picture. Serum chromium is difficult to measure reliably, but dietary assessment for refined sugar intake provides a functional proxy. 25(OH)D alongside PTH and magnesium provides the vitamin D functional picture.

The information in this chapter is educational and does not constitute clinical advice. The management of thyroid disease, diabetes, and other endocrine conditions requires individualized clinical assessment. In particular, selenium supplementation in Hashimoto's thyroiditis should be discussed with an endocrinologist or treating physician, as it has documented clinical evidence in some protocols but requires professional oversight regarding dose and duration. The author does not offer clinical recommendations for any individual.

IX. James's Orchestra, Reconsidered

James has been on levothyroxine for six years. His TSH is in range. His selenium has never been measured. His free T3 has been measured once in six years and was in the low-normal range — a finding documented and not acted upon. His zinc has never been measured. His iron status was checked at diagnosis and not since. His anti-TPO antibodies were noted at diagnosis and have been monitored but not addressed nutritionally. His vitamin D was low-normal at last check and a supplement was recommended; whether he is taking it has not been followed up.

The orchestra of his thyroid system is playing with at least five musicians absent or performing below capacity. The TSH measurement — the single note that determines whether his medication is adjusted — is the sound of the one musician that the medication has replaced. The rest of the orchestra is silent. And nobody is listening for it.

For the Clinically Curious

Deiodinase Enzymes — The Selenium-Dependent Conversion System

Three deiodinase isoenzymes regulate thyroid hormone activation and inactivation. Type I deiodinase (DIO1) in the liver and kidney performs the primary T4→T3 conversion in the circulation. Type II deiodinase (DIO2) in the brain, pituitary, and other tissues provides local T3 production for tissue-specific needs. Type III deiodinase (DIO3) inactivates T3 and T4 by converting them to rT3 (reverse T3) and T2 respectively. All three are selenoproteins, containing selenocysteine at their active sites. Under conditions of selenium deficiency, DIO1 activity is preferentially reduced while DIO3 activity is maintained — resulting in a shift toward rT3 production at the expense of active T3. Elevated reverse T3 relative to T3 — not a standard component of routine thyroid function testing — may indicate selenium insufficiency as a component of impaired T4 utilization.

Chromodulin and the Insulin Signaling Cascade

Chromodulin (historically called low-molecular-weight chromium-binding substance or LMWCr) is an oligopeptide containing four chromium (III) atoms that is released from liver and kidney in response to insulin stimulation. Chromodulin binds to the activated (insulin-bound) insulin receptor and amplifies its autophosphorylation activity by approximately eight-fold, potentiating insulin signaling downstream. The mechanism is distinct from insulin receptor kinase activity and represents a chromium-specific amplification step. Clinical trials of chromium supplementation in type 2 diabetes have produced mixed results, reflecting the heterogeneity of chromium status in study populations. Meta-analyses of better-controlled studies consistently show significant improvements in fasting glucose, HbA1c, and insulin sensitivity — particularly in chromium-insufficient populations.

Selenium and Anti-TPO Antibodies — The Clinical Evidence

A systematic review and meta-analysis published in Thyroid (2018) pooled data from eleven randomized controlled trials of selenium supplementation in Hashimoto's thyroiditis and found significant reductions in anti-TPO antibody titres (weighted mean difference approximately -40 IU/mL, $p<0.001$) at three and six months compared to placebo. The evidence for anti-TG antibody reduction is more mixed. The mechanism involves selenoprotein-mediated reduction of hydrogen peroxide in thyroid follicular cells: DIO1, glutathione peroxidase, and thioredoxin reductase — all selenoproteins — collectively reduce the oxidative burden in thyroid tissue that generates the neoepitopes driving antibody production. Selenium supplementation in Hashimoto's is not yet part of standard endocrinology guidelines in most countries, despite a consistency of evidence that would be considered actionable if it involved a pharmaceutical compound.

The Magnesium-Insulin Resistance Loop

Intracellular magnesium is required for insulin receptor tyrosine kinase activity. In insulin resistance, intracellular magnesium is reduced — partly because insulin-stimulated magnesium uptake is impaired, creating a state in which impaired insulin signaling reduces magnesium uptake which further impairs insulin signaling. This bidirectional reinforcing relationship is supported by multiple lines of evidence: prospective cohort studies consistently find inverse relationships between magnesium intake and incident type 2 diabetes (approximately 15% risk reduction per 100mg/day increment); clinical trials show significant improvements in insulin sensitivity with magnesium supplementation in hypomagnesemic subjects; and serum magnesium is significantly lower in diabetic patients than matched controls independent of dietary intake, reflecting the intracellular depletion of RBC magnesium that is not captured by the serum measurement.

Cluster 7

The Neurological Foundations

How Twelve Nutrients Power and Protect the Brain and Nervous System — and Why Depression, Cognitive Decline, and Neurological Disease Are Being Medicated Without Ever Asking What the Brain Is Running On

> *"The brain is not immune to the laws of biochemistry. It is the most biochemically demanding organ in the body. Feed it poorly and it thinks poorly. Deplete it of its essential nutrients and it begins to fail, quietly, over years, in ways that look like diseases with names and none of those names is 'nutritional insufficiency'."*

I. The Most Expensive Orchestra Section

Sarah is thirty-eight years old. She has been treated for major depression for four years with two different antidepressants. The second has provided meaningful relief from the deepest darkness

— the kind that made mornings impossible. But a persistent fog remains. Her memory, which was sharp before the depression, has not returned to its previous standard. She is motivated but sluggish. Her psychiatrist has suggested augmentation with a second pharmacological agent.

In four years of treatment, nobody has measured her serum B12. Nobody has assessed her folate status, her methylmalonic acid, her plasma homocysteine. Nobody has measured her omega-3 index — the EPA and DHA content of her red blood cell membranes, which reflects the fatty acid composition of the neuronal membranes through which every serotonin signal travels. Nobody has checked her iron, despite the fact that iron is a required cofactor for tryptophan hydroxylase, the first enzyme in serotonin synthesis. Nobody has assessed her zinc, which modulates the BDNF signaling that drives the neuroplasticity on which antidepressant treatment partly depends.

Sarah's treatment has been directed entirely at the downstream chemistry of a system whose upstream nutritional substrate is entirely opaque to everyone managing her care. The orchestra is playing poorly. The instruments are being tuned at the far end of the hall. Nobody has walked back to where the musicians sit.

II. Meet the Cast

Twelve musicians comprise the neurological orchestra described in this chapter. Together they supply energy to neurons, synthesize the neurotransmitters that govern mood and cognition, maintain the myelin sheaths that enable nerve conduction, protect neurons from oxidative damage, and regulate the signaling systems through which the brain responds to experience and adapts over time.

- **Thiamine (B1)** — Primary energy supplier to neurons via the Krebs cycle gateway. Also the cofactor for alpha-ketoglutarate dehydrogenase, whose impairment disrupts neurotransmitter precursor balance and produces neurological symptoms before frank beriberi is evident.
- **Niacin (B3) and NAD+** — NAD+ is the primary electron carrier for neuronal energy production and the substrate for PARP enzymes that repair damaged neuronal DNA. Pellagra — niacin deficiency — produces psychosis, dementia, and depression before the skin manifestations appear.
- **Vitamin B6 (Pyridoxal-5-Phosphate)** — Cofactor for the decarboxylase enzymes that produce serotonin, dopamine, GABA, noradrenaline, and taurine. Without B6, neurotransmitter synthesis stalls at the penultimate step regardless of amino acid substrate availability.
- **Vitamin B12 (Methylcobalamin)** — Required for myelin synthesis, methylation of neuronal DNA, and regeneration of methionine from homocysteine via methionine synthase. Deficiency produces subacute combined degeneration of the spinal cord — a demyelinating condition indistinguishable from copper deficiency myelopathy in its early stages.

- **Folate (Methylfolate)** — Required for one-carbon metabolism in neuronal DNA synthesis and methylation. Provides the methyl group that drives methionine synthase. The MTHFR C677T variant impairs folate conversion to its active methylfolate form, connecting genetic variation to neurological nutritional vulnerability.
- **Choline** — Precursor to acetylcholine — the neurotransmitter of learning, memory, and parasympathetic function. Also the structural head group of phosphatidylcholine, the dominant phospholipid in neuronal membranes. Choline demand is highest during fetal brain development and in aging brains losing cholinergic neurons.
- **Omega-3 fatty acids — EPA and DHA** — DHA constitutes approximately sixty percent of the brain's structural fat and dominates neuronal synaptic membranes. EPA modulates neuroinflammation. Together they determine membrane fluidity, receptor conformational dynamics, and the physical efficiency of every synaptic transaction in the brain.
- **Zinc** — Required for BDNF (brain-derived neurotrophic factor) receptor signaling, NMDA receptor modulation, and zinc-finger transcription factors regulating neuronal gene expression. Rapidly depleted by psychological stress. Its insufficiency impairs the neuroplasticity on which antidepressant treatment and cognitive recovery depend.
- **Magnesium** — The physiological blocker of NMDA receptors at rest — preventing the calcium influx that would otherwise produce neuronal excitotoxicity under baseline conditions. Magnesium deficiency removes this protective block, producing anxiety, pain hypersensitivity, insomnia, and

migraine through a mechanistically specific neurochemical pathway.

- **Iron** — Required for the hydroxylase enzymes that convert tryptophan to serotonin and tyrosine to dopamine. Also required for myelination — iron deficiency in infancy produces irreversible reductions in dopamine receptor density and cognitive capacity. Iron-deficiency anemia is the most common nutritional deficiency in children globally and a preventable cause of cognitive impairment.
- **Lithium (trace)** — At trace dietary amounts far below therapeutic doses for bipolar disorder, lithium inhibits GSK-3 beta, upregulates BDNF, modulates neuroinflammation, and may be neuroprotective. Ecological studies consistently show inverse correlations between drinking water lithium concentrations and rates of suicide, dementia, and violent crime at the population level.
- **Vitamin D** — A neurosteroid whose receptors are expressed throughout the brain — particularly in the hippocampus and prefrontal cortex. Regulates neurotrophin synthesis, modulates neuroinflammation, and is inversely associated with depression, schizophrenia, and cognitive decline in population studies.

These twelve musicians produce the substrate of thought, emotion, memory, and neurological function. Their collective sufficiency determines not simply whether the brain works — it does, across a wide range of nutritional states — but how well it works, how resilient it is, how completely it recovers from disruption, and how gracefully it ages.

III. The Neurotransmitter Production Line

Serotonin — The Iron-B6 Chain

Serotonin is synthesized from tryptophan in two enzymatic steps. Tryptophan hydroxylase — the first and rate-limiting enzyme — requires iron as a cofactor and converts tryptophan to 5-hydroxytryptophan (5-HTP). Aromatic amino acid decarboxylase — the second enzyme — requires pyridoxal-5-phosphate (active vitamin B6) and converts 5-HTP to serotonin. Both steps can be impaired by the relevant nutrient insufficiency independently of each other and independently of the SSRIs that prevent serotonin's reuptake. An SSRI prescribed to a patient with iron deficiency or B6 insufficiency is acting on the downstream availability of a neurotransmitter whose upstream production is impaired — producing partial responses that are attributed to the medication's limits rather than to the substrate problem it cannot address.

Tryptophan's brain entry adds another layer of complexity. It crosses the blood-brain barrier via the large neutral amino acid (LNAA) transporter — sharing that transporter with leucine, isoleucine, valine, phenylalanine, and tyrosine. The brain uptake of tryptophan is determined not by its absolute plasma concentration but by its ratio to these competing amino acids. A high-protein meal rich in branched-chain amino acids can paradoxically reduce brain tryptophan uptake and serotonin synthesis despite adequate dietary tryptophan, because competition at the transporter limits entry.

Dopamine — The Catecholamine Cascade

The catecholamine synthesis chain — from tyrosine through L-DOPA, dopamine, noradrenaline, and adrenaline — requires four separate nutrients at successive enzymatic steps. Tyrosine hydroxylase requires iron and a tetrahydrobiopterin cofactor to convert tyrosine to L-DOPA. Aromatic amino acid decarboxylase (B6-dependent) converts L-DOPA to dopamine. Dopamine beta-hydroxylase — a copper enzyme that also requires vitamin C — converts dopamine to noradrenaline. Phenylethanolamine N-methyltransferase (SAMe-dependent, connecting the methylation network) produces adrenaline from noradrenaline.

The clinical implications are profound and consistently overlooked. A patient with ADHD, depression, Parkinson's disease, or any condition characterized by dopaminergic insufficiency has an upstream catecholamine production system that depends on adequate iron, B6, copper, and vitamin C at successive steps. The medication prescribed to adjust dopamine signaling does not address the production chain upstream of it. Measuring and addressing these upstream nutritional inputs alongside pharmaceutical management is not alternative medicine — it is completing the biochemical picture that the drug acts on.

GABA — The B6 Brake

GABA is the brain's primary inhibitory neurotransmitter. It is produced from glutamate by glutamate decarboxylase — an enzyme that requires pyridoxal-5-phosphate (active B6) as its essential cofactor. Without adequate B6, the conversion of glutamate to GABA is impaired, the brain's excitatory-inhibitory balance shifts toward excitation, and the neurochemical substrate for anxiety, seizure susceptibility, insomnia, and pain hypersensitivity is created.

This B6-GABA connection is one of the most direct nutrient-neurotransmitter relationships in the brain and one of the most clinically consequential — yet it is essentially absent from psychiatric and neurological practice. Benzodiazepines that enhance GABA receptor sensitivity, and the anticonvulsants that modulate GABAergic tone, are prescribed without any assessment of the B6 status that determines the baseline availability of GABA itself. The drug adjusts the receptor's response to GABA. The nutrient determines how much GABA is available to act on that receptor.

IV. Myelin — The Insulation B12 and Copper Protect

Myelin is the fatty sheath surrounding neuronal axons that enables rapid electrical signal propagation. Without myelin, nerve signals travel slowly and with significant signal loss. Demyelinating diseases — multiple sclerosis, subacute combined degeneration, peripheral neuropathies — are characterized by the loss of this insulation and the resulting failure of rapid, precise neural conduction.

Vitamin B12 is required for myelin synthesis through its role in the methylation cycle (methylmalonyl-CoA mutase converts methylmalonyl-CoA to succinyl-CoA; its failure leads to accumulation of odd-chain fatty acids incorporated into myelin abnormally) and through its support of the methionine cycle that provides the methyl groups for myelin membrane phospholipid synthesis. Classical B12 deficiency produces subacute combined degeneration of the spinal cord — T2 hyperintensity in the dorsal and lateral columns on MRI, progressive sensory loss, weakness, and balance impairment.

Copper deficiency produces an identical clinical and MRI picture — frequently misdiagnosed as B12 deficiency or multiple sclerosis because copper measurement is not reflexively included in neurological workups. The two conditions — both producing demyelinating myelopathy — require measurement of both nutrients for accurate diagnosis. One is routinely checked. The other almost never is.

DHA constitutes approximately sixty percent of myelin's lipid content. The quality of the lipid in which myelin proteins are embedded affects myelin function just as the quality of insulation on an electrical cable affects conduction. An omega-3-depleted diet producing DHA-poor neuronal and myelin membranes creates a neural signaling environment that is structurally less efficient than one built on adequate DHA — not dramatically enough to produce a diagnosable demyelinating condition, but sufficiently to impair the speed and precision of neural transmission throughout the brain and nervous system.

V. The Brain's Membrane — DHA and the Architecture of Thought

Approximately sixty percent of the brain's dry weight is fat. Of this, DHA — docosahexaenoic acid — is the single most abundant fatty acid in synaptic membranes, the sites where every neurotransmitter signal is sent and received. DHA's structural dominance in these membranes is not incidental. It is functional. The physical properties of the membrane — how fluid it is, how quickly its proteins can move and change conformation, how efficiently its ion channels open and close — depend on DHA content.

DHA-rich membranes are more fluid. Fluid membranes enable faster receptor conformational changes when neurotransmitters bind. Faster conformational changes mean more rapid and more efficient synaptic transmission. The neurotransmitter molecules that SSRIs, antipsychotics, and anxiolytics act on reside in membranes whose physical properties are determined by the DHA content of the diet over the preceding months. A medication that modulates a receptor's behavior is acting on a receptor embedded in a membrane whose physical environment has never been characterized.

The omega-3 index — EPA and DHA as a percentage of total red blood cell fatty acids — directly reflects the DHA content of cell membranes body-wide, including neuronal membranes. Western populations average an omega-3 index of four to five percent. Populations eating traditional diets rich in fatty fish consistently show indexes of eight percent or above. The difference between these values is a measurable difference in neuronal membrane composition — a difference whose consequences for mood, cognition, and neurological function are documented across hundreds of population studies and clinical trials.

VI. The NMDA Receptor — Where Magnesium Protects

The NMDA receptor is both the primary mechanism of synaptic plasticity — the molecular basis of learning and memory — and a potential site of excitotoxic neuronal death when inappropriately activated. At rest, a magnesium ion physically blocks the NMDA receptor's ion channel. The channel opens only when two conditions are simultaneously met: the receiving neuron is sufficiently depolarised AND glutamate binds the receptor. This coincidence-detection mechanism — Hebbian learning at the molecular level — is what makes NMDA receptors the basis of associative memory.

When magnesium is insufficient, the resting block is reduced or absent. The NMDA receptor becomes more easily activated by ambient glutamate under baseline conditions. The result is increased background neuronal excitability — a neurochemical correlate of anxiety, hypervigilance, pain sensitivity, and the sleep-initiation difficulty that characterizes anxiety-related insomnia. This mechanism is pharmacologically precise: the drug ketamine acts as an NMDA receptor antagonist, and its rapid antidepressant effect is thought to derive partly from restoring NMDA receptor regulation. Magnesium performs the physiological version of the same function. The distinction is that magnesium insufficiency is common, measurable, addressable, and essentially never investigated in the psychiatric management of anxiety and insomnia.

VII. The Web of Dependencies

B12 requires folate: Methionine synthase — the B12-dependent enzyme that regenerates methionine and enables myelin synthesis — requires methylfolate as its methyl donor. B12 and folate are metabolically inseparable. Supplementing B12 without folate, or folate without B12, produces incomplete neurological recovery.

Serotonin requires iron and B6: Tryptophan hydroxylase (iron) and aromatic amino acid decarboxylase (B6) are both required for serotonin synthesis. An SSRI cannot improve serotonin availability in a patient with iron deficiency or B6 insufficiency because the synthesis pipeline that the drug's reuptake inhibition depends on is producing less serotonin to begin with.

DHA requires vitamin E: DHA is highly polyunsaturated and vulnerable to lipid peroxidation. Vitamin E — the membrane-resident antioxidant — protects DHA in neuronal membranes from oxidative damage. A brain that is DHA-replete but vitamin E-depleted has the right structural fatty acid but inadequate protection for it.

Magnesium requires vitamin D for absorption: Vitamin D upregulates the intestinal transporter for magnesium absorption. In vitamin D-deficient states, dietary magnesium is less efficiently absorbed — contributing to the magnesium insufficiency that impairs NMDA receptor regulation, ATP activation, and neurotransmitter synthesis simultaneously.

Trace lithium requires adequate dietary provision: Unlike other nutrients in this chapter, lithium cannot be synthesized by the body and has no reliable food source that provides consistent amounts — its concentration in plant foods varies with soil geology. In geological regions with low lithium in groundwater and soil, dietary lithium may be consistently below the trace amounts associated with neuroprotective effects in population studies.

> *Sarah's antidepressant adjusts the downstream availability of serotonin whose upstream synthesis requires iron and B6 it has never had measured, in a*

> *neuronal membrane composed of DHA whose status in her cells has never been assessed, modulating BDNF signaling that requires zinc whose level in her body is unknown, in a brain whose NMDA receptor protection by magnesium has never been evaluated, through a methylation cycle whose efficiency depends on folate, B12, and riboflavin that have never been optimized. The partial response is not a medication failure. It is the predictable arithmetic of treating one variable in a system with twelve.*

VIII. Questions Worth Asking

For a person with depression, anxiety, poor memory, cognitive fog, neuropathy, balance difficulty, or neurological symptoms that have not fully responded to pharmaceutical management — the neurological nutrient network is an upstream territory that is assessable, measurable, and rarely systematically explored.

Serum B12 is a poor functional marker — it may be normal while cellular B12 deficiency exists. Methylmalonic acid (MMA) in plasma or urine is the functional marker that reveals B12 insufficiency at the cellular level when serum B12 appears adequate. Plasma homocysteine elevates in B12, folate, and B6 insufficiency and is itself neurotoxic at elevated concentrations. RBC folate alongside plasma folate provides a picture of longer-term folate status.

Plasma omega-3 index (EPA+DHA as percentage of RBC fatty acids) directly measures neuronal membrane fatty acid composition. Serum zinc alongside alkaline phosphatase (a zinc-dependent enzyme whose low activity indicates functional zinc insufficiency). RBC magnesium, not serum magnesium. Serum ferritin alongside transferrin saturation and CRP (distinguishing iron deficiency from iron sequestration in inflammation). 25(OH)D alongside PTH and magnesium.

The information in this chapter is educational and does not constitute clinical or psychiatric advice. The management of depression, anxiety, and other neurological and psychiatric conditions requires professional diagnosis and is not replaced by nutritional assessment or supplementation. The nutritional factors described here are potentially complementary to appropriate professional care and are worth discussing with a qualified healthcare professional. The author does not offer clinical recommendations for any individual.

IX. Sarah's Orchestra, Reconsidered

Sarah's four years of antidepressant treatment have addressed one variable in a twelve-variable system. Her serum B12 has never been measured. Her methylmalonic acid has never been checked. Her plasma folate is in range — but the active methylfolate form that crosses her blood-brain barrier has never been assessed, and her MTHFR status has never been tested. Her omega-3 index has never been measured. Her zinc is unknown. Her magnesium has never been assessed beyond a standard serum panel that would appear normal even with significant intracellular depletion. Her iron was checked once, three years ago, and was low-normal.

The partial response that has frustrated her treatment — the lifted darkness that did not become full restoration — is not the medication's ceiling. It is the consequence of treating one instrument in a twelve-piece section. The serotonin reuptake inhibitor is performing its function. The synthesis pipeline it depends on, the membrane it signals through, the BDNF it co-activates, the homocysteine load that the methylation system is placing on her neurological chemistry — none of it has been assessed. None of it has been addressed. The full orchestra is playing short-staffed, and the sound that reaches the audience is called a partial responder.

For the Clinically Curious

MTHFR and Neuropsychiatric Risk — The Methylation-Neurotransmitter Connection

The MTHFR C677T polymorphism reduces methylfolate production, impairing the methionine synthase reaction and elevating homocysteine. In the CNS, reduced methylfolate availability impairs the methylation of biopterin precursors required for tetrahydrobiopterin (BH4) synthesis. BH4 is an obligate cofactor for tryptophan hydroxylase (serotonin synthesis) and tyrosine hydroxylase (dopamine/noradrenaline synthesis). A methylation network impaired by MTHFR variants, B12 insufficiency, or folate depletion therefore reduces neurotransmitter synthesis capacity through BH4 depletion — a mechanism entirely independent of the reuptake inhibition targeted by SSRI and SNRI medications. Methylfolate supplementation — bypassing the impaired MTHFR step — has been studied as an adjunct to SSRI treatment in C677T carriers and has shown significant improvements in treatment response in this genotype-specific subgroup. This represents one of the clearest examples in psychiatry of a genetically defined nutritional intervention that the field has not yet integrated into standard practice.

Lithium at Trace Dietary Levels — Population Evidence and Mechanism

Epidemiological studies across multiple countries (Japan, USA, Austria, Greece, UK, Lithuania) have consistently found inverse correlations between naturally occurring lithium concentrations in drinking water (range 0.1–200 μg/L) and rates of suicide, homicide, and violent crime. A 2018 meta-analysis of

27 studies found a pooled significant inverse correlation. At trace levels, lithium inhibits glycogen synthase kinase-3 beta (GSK-3β) — a kinase whose overactivity is implicated in bipolar disorder, Alzheimer's disease, and treatment-resistant depression — and upregulates BDNF through CREB phosphorylation. The neurotrophin effect and GSK-3β inhibition at trace doses are distinct from the sodium channel effects and mood stabilization at therapeutic doses (600–1800 mg/day lithium carbonate). Dietary trace lithium intake from food and water averages 0.4–3 mg/day in most populations; residents of high-lithium geological regions consume several-fold more from water alone. The neuroprotective relevance of chronic trace lithium insufficiency in low-lithium geological regions is biologically plausible but not yet translated into clinical recommendations.

Copper Deficiency Myelopathy — The Neurological Diagnosis Medicine Misses

Copper deficiency myelopathy (CDM) presents as progressive sensorimotor dysfunction with T2 hyperintensity in the posterior and lateral columns of the cervical and thoracic spinal cord on MRI — radiologically and clinically indistinguishable from B12 deficiency subacute combined degeneration of the spinal cord. Causes include: zinc supplementation (the most common Western cause — high zinc saturates metallothionein and prevents copper absorption), gastric bypass surgery, celiac disease, inflammatory bowel disease, and prolonged use of zinc-containing denture adhesives (multiple published case series). A 2010 systematic review identified over 50 published CDM cases initially misdiagnosed as MS or idiopathic myelopathy before copper measurement identified the cause. Standard neurological workup for progressive myelopathy rarely includes serum copper, ceruloplasmin, and RBC copper as a matter of course — a gap that results in delayed diagnosis and treatment while neurological damage progresses. Copper replenishment halts CDM progression in most cases; reversal of existing deficits is partial and depends on duration.

Magnesium and the NMDA Receptor — Clinical Translation

The voltage-dependent Mg2+ block of the NMDA receptor channel requires extracellular Mg2+ concentrations in the millimolar range for physiologically relevant blocking. Cerebrospinal fluid magnesium is maintained at approximately 1.0–1.2 mmol/L (slightly higher than plasma). Multiple clinical conditions associated with magnesium depletion — including migraine, anxiety disorders, fibromyalgia, and chronic pain syndromes — are characterized by NMDA receptor hyperactivation. A 2017 randomized controlled trial (Limonie et al., PLOS One) found that magnesium glycinate supplementation at 248 mg/day significantly reduced depression and anxiety scores in mildly to moderately deficient adults. A 2016 review of 18 studies found consistent associations between low magnesium status and depression. The mechanistic basis — impaired Mg2+ NMDA receptor block, increased cortisol-driven Mg2+ excretion under stress, and reduced serotonin synthesis from Mg2+-requiring enzyme steps — provides a coherent upstream rationale that has not been integrated into first-line psychiatric management.

Cluster 8

The Immune Architects

How Ten Nutrients Build, Calibrate, and Restrain the Immune System — and Why Autoimmune Disease, Chronic Infection, and Cancer Risk Are Conditions Medicine Treats Without Looking at the Blueprint That Built Them

> *"The immune system does not turn against itself at random. It turns against itself when it has not been given the conditions it needs to learn the difference between self and enemy. Those conditions are nutritional."*

I. The Army Built on Minerals

Priya is forty-six years old. She has had rheumatoid arthritis for eight years, managed with a biological agent that suppresses TNF-alpha — one of the primary inflammatory cytokines driving her joint destruction. The treatment has been effective at slowing structural damage. Her joint swelling has reduced. Her X-rays are stable. She remains functionally impaired, fatigued, and prone to infections.

She is told this is the expected profile of managed rheumatoid arthritis.

Nobody has asked about the nutritional conditions that produced an immune system willing to attack the synovial membrane of her own joints. Nobody has measured her vitamin D, which governs the development of the regulatory T-cells whose job is to prevent exactly this kind of immune self-targeting. Nobody has considered her omega-3 status, which determines whether the prostaglandins driving her joint inflammation can be resolved by adequate EPA-derived resolvins. Nobody has assessed her zinc, required for every immune cell type's development and function. Nobody has looked at her gut microbiome — the ecosystem that programs regulatory immune circuits from birth and whose disruption creates the permissive environment for autoimmunity.

The biological agent Priya receives is a remarkable pharmacological achievement. It suppresses one cytokine at the downstream end of an immune cascade that begins somewhere upstream in the ecology of her immune system. That upstream ecology — nutritional, microbial, endocrine, inflammatory — has never been the focus of her treatment.

II. Meet the Cast

Ten musicians comprise the immune orchestra described in this chapter. Together they govern the development of immune cells in the thymus and bone marrow, the calibration of immune responses between defense and tolerance, the maintenance of the regulatory circuits that prevent autoimmunity, and the resolution of inflammation when the immune system's work is done.

- **Vitamin D** — The master immune modulator. Acts through vitamin D receptors expressed on virtually every immune cell type — suppressing Th1 and Th17 (autoimmune-prone) responses and promoting regulatory T-cell development. The most consistent nutritional correlate of autoimmune disease susceptibility.
- **Zinc** — Required for the development and maturation of every immune cell type. Thymulin — the thymic hormone that enables T-cell maturation — requires zinc at its active site and is biologically inactive without it. Zinc deficiency produces thymic atrophy and T-cell lymphopenia.
- **Selenium** — Required for glutathione peroxidase and thioredoxin reductase in immune cells — protecting immune cells from the oxidative burst they generate when killing pathogens. Also governs the balance between pro-inflammatory and anti-inflammatory immune responses.
- **Vitamin A** — The guardian of mucosal immunity — governs goblet cell differentiation, mucin production, and secretory IgA synthesis at the gut, respiratory, and urogenital mucosal surfaces. Deficiency impairs the first line of immune defense before any systemic immune response is required.
- **Vitamin C** — Consumed in large quantities by neutrophils during the oxidative burst that kills bacteria. Required for T-cell proliferation, antibody production, and the regeneration

of glutathione that protects immune cells from their own oxidative weapons.

- **Iron** — Required for the rapid proliferation of immune cells during an active immune response — immune cell division demands adequate iron for DNA synthesis. Also the cofactor for myeloperoxidase, the enzyme that generates the hypochlorite used in the bactericidal oxidative burst.
- **Omega-3 fatty acids — EPA** — The precursor to the E-series resolvins and anti-inflammatory prostaglandin E3. EPA competes with arachidonic acid for the same enzymatic pathways, shifting the balance from inflammatory amplification toward inflammatory resolution. The omega-3:omega-6 ratio determines whether the immune system can complete the termination of inflammation or sustains it chronically.
- **Magnesium** — Required for LFA-1 integrin function on cytotoxic T-cells — the molecular anchor that allows T-cells to bind and kill their targets. In 2022, a landmark Cell paper demonstrated that magnesium deficiency impairs the cytotoxic function of T-cells against cancer cells through this LFA-1 mechanism.
- **Glutamine** — The primary fuel for rapidly proliferating immune cells during an acute immune response. Immune cell glutamine demand during infection or surgery can deplete systemic glutamine reserves, impairing the immune response's endurance and the gut barrier integrity that determines how much bacterial translocation the immune system must manage.

- **Glycine** — An inhibitory modulator of macrophage and neutrophil NF-κB activation — directly reducing pro-inflammatory cytokine production in the most inflammatory immune cells. Anti-inflammatory at the molecular level independent of its structural roles in collagen and glutathione.

These ten musicians together determine whether the immune system can mount an adequate defense, calibrate it appropriately, complete it when the threat is eliminated, and maintain the tolerogenic state that prevents autoimmune self-targeting. Each insufficiency moves the immune system's operating point — toward immunosuppression, toward inflammatory excess, toward autoimmune permissiveness, or toward impaired resolution. The position of that operating point is largely determined by the ten nutrients in this chapter.

III. How the Immune System Is Organized

The Innate Response — Fast, Non-Specific, Nutrient-Hungry

The innate immune system responds to infection within minutes. Neutrophils — the most abundant white blood cells, produced in the bone marrow at a rate of approximately 100 billion per day — are the first responders. They migrate to sites of infection, engulf pathogens through phagocytosis, and kill them through two primary mechanisms: the oxidative burst (generating hypochlorite, hydrogen peroxide, and superoxide from iron-containing myeloperoxidase) and degranulation (releasing stored antimicrobial proteins). Both mechanisms are nutrient-dependent. The oxidative burst requires iron and consumes vitamin C stoichiometrically — neutrophil vitamin C concentration is among the highest in any tissue, and it drops rapidly during an acute infection.

Natural killer (NK) cells recognize virus-infected and tumor cells through surface receptor patterns and kill them by releasing cytotoxic granules. NK cell function requires selenium and zinc for the enzyme systems that regulate their killing capacity. Vitamin D upregulates NK cell cytotoxicity. Iron deficiency reduces NK cell numbers. The entire innate response — rapid, non-specific, first-line — depends on the ten musicians described in this chapter.

The Adaptive Response — Slow, Precise, Memory-Building

The adaptive immune response develops over days to weeks, generating targeted lymphocytes whose specificity is matched to a particular pathogen. T-lymphocytes mature in the thymus through a process that requires zinc (for thymulin activity), vitamin D (for T-cell differentiation signals), and adequate antioxidant protection (selenium, vitamin C) for the high-division cells. B-lymphocytes producing antibodies require iron, zinc, and vitamin C for the rapid proliferation of the clonal expansion phase. The memory cells generated after a successful immune response — the cellular basis of lasting immunity — are maintained by vitamin D, zinc, and selenium over the months and years between exposures.

Regulatory T-Cells — The Immune Brake

Regulatory T-cells (Tregs) are the immune system's primary autoimmunity prevention mechanism. They develop in the gut-associated lymphoid tissue under the instruction of specific gut bacteria and under the direct influence of vitamin D. Their master transcription factor — Foxp3 — is directly upregulated by 1,25-dihydroxyvitamin D3 through VDR signaling. Butyrate from gut bacterial fermentation of dietary fiber also drives Foxp3 expression through HDAC inhibition. Vitamin A, through its RXR-VDR receptor interactions, co-activates the vitamin D signal that promotes Treg differentiation.

The modern conditions for autoimmunity are largely the conditions that deplete regulatory T-cell development: vitamin D deficiency (impaired Foxp3 induction), gut dysbiosis (impaired butyrate production and microbial Treg education), low-fiber diets (reduced butyrate substrate), and excess omega-6 fatty acids (producing the prostaglandin E2 that suppresses Treg development). These conditions describe the lifestyle profile of a large proportion of modern Western populations. They describe Priya's profile with precision.

IV. Vitamin D — The Master Calibrator

The vitamin D receptor (VDR) is expressed in every immune cell type that has been examined. 1,25-dihydroxyvitamin D3 binding to

VDR produces a predominantly tolerogenic immune phenotype: suppression of Th1 cytokines (IFN-gamma, IL-12) that drive autoimmune attack, suppression of Th17 cells that drive inflammatory tissue destruction, promotion of Th2 and regulatory T-cell differentiation, reduction of NF-κB inflammatory signaling, and upregulation of antimicrobial peptides (defensins and cathelicidins) that provide direct pathogen killing without inflammatory activation.

The epidemiological evidence for vitamin D's role in autoimmune disease is among the most consistent in nutritional epidemiology. Multiple sclerosis prevalence increases with latitude (lower UV, lower vitamin D) in every country where data are available. Rheumatoid arthritis, inflammatory bowel disease, type 1 diabetes, systemic lupus erythematosus, and psoriasis all show inverse associations with vitamin D status in population studies. Genome-wide association studies identify VDR polymorphisms as susceptibility factors across multiple autoimmune conditions. Intervention trials with vitamin D supplementation have shown reductions in anti-nuclear antibody titres, improvements in disease activity scores in multiple sclerosis, and significant reductions in new autoimmune disease diagnosis in primary prevention populations.

Priya's rheumatoid arthritis is a Th1 and Th17-dominant autoimmune condition — precisely the immune phenotype that vitamin D, mechanistically, is positioned to moderate. Her vitamin D status has never been systematically targeted as part of her rheumatological management. The biological agent suppresses

TNF-alpha downstream of the Th1/Th17 activation that adequate vitamin D might reduce upstream.

V. The Omega-3:Omega-6 Ratio and Inflammatory Resolution

Inflammation is not simply a problem to be suppressed. It is a physiological process with two phases: initiation and resolution. The initiation phase — the recruitment of neutrophils, the production of prostaglandins and leukotrienes, the activation of macrophages — is necessary for killing pathogens and clearing damaged tissue. The resolution phase — the clearance of cellular debris, the suppression of further recruitment, the restoration of tissue homeostasis — is equally necessary and equally active. Inflammation that resolves is beneficial. Inflammation that does not resolve is chronic disease.

The molecules that drive resolution — the E-series resolvins (from EPA), the D-series resolvins and protectins (from DHA), and the lipoxins (from arachidonic acid) — are biosynthesized from polyunsaturated fatty acids. Their production depends on adequate EPA and DHA in cell membranes. With the modern dietary omega-3:omega-6 ratio of approximately 15:1, cell membranes are dominated by arachidonic acid, which is converted preferentially to pro-inflammatory PGE2 and LTB4. The resolution mediators cannot be produced at adequate levels because their substrates — EPA and DHA — are proportionally scarce.

Priya's joint inflammation may not resolve efficiently between flares because the resolution biology — the EPA-derived E-series resolvins that would actively terminate inflammation and clear the joint debris — is being outcompeted at every enzymatic step by arachidonic acid. This is not a diagnosis. It is a metabolic state measurable with a simple RBC fatty acid profile. It is addressable with dietary change and EPA supplementation. It has never been the focus of her rheumatological treatment.

VI. Magnesium and T-Cell Killing — The 2022 Discovery

In 2022, a paper published in Cell described a previously unrecognized magnesium-T-cell dependency with direct implications for cancer immunology and immune defense. LFA-1 (lymphocyte function-associated antigen 1) is the integrin on the surface of cytotoxic T-cells and NK cells that enables them to form the immunological synapse — the contact point with a target cell (tumor cell or virus-infected cell) through which cytotoxic granules are delivered.

LFA-1 requires magnesium to adopt its high-affinity binding conformation. In magnesium-depleted environments — including the magnesium-poor microenvironment of many solid tumors — LFA-1 cannot engage efficiently, the immunological synapse is impaired, and cytotoxic killing is reduced. The functional consequence is that T-cells attempting to kill cancer cells in a low-magnesium environment are less effective regardless of their numbers and their activation state.

The clinical implication is significant: the widespread magnesium insufficiency of modern populations may be impairing T-cell and NK cell cytotoxic function against nascent tumor cells throughout the body on a continuous basis. This is not the same as a diagnosable immune deficiency. It is a subtle but continuous reduction in the immune surveillance that prevents tumor cells from establishing themselves before they reach clinical detection. Magnesium is cheap, measurable, and correctable. Its role in T-cell cytotoxic function has been established at the molecular level. The clinical translation — assessing magnesium status as a component of cancer prevention and immunological support — has yet to find its way into mainstream medical practice.

VII. The Web of Dependencies

Vitamin D requires magnesium: Both hydroxylation steps that convert vitamin D to its active form — in the liver (25-hydroxylation) and in the kidney (1-alpha-hydroxylation) — are catalyzed by magnesium-dependent hydroxylases. In magnesium-depleted states, supplemental vitamin D raises 25(OH)D but fails to produce the full immunological effect that requires adequate 1,25(OH)2D production.

Zinc and copper balance: High-dose zinc supplementation — widely used for immune support — suppresses copper absorption through metallothionein competition. Copper is required for neutrophil production and function, for superoxide dismutase activity in immune cells, and for lysyl oxidase in the collagen structures of lymphoid organs. The immune benefit of zinc supplementation may be partially offset by the immune cost of copper depletion if the two minerals are not balanced.

Selenium and vitamin E: Glutathione peroxidase (selenium-dependent) protects immune cell membranes from the oxidative damage generated during immune activation. Vitamin E is the membrane antioxidant partner — after vitamin E neutralizes a lipid peroxyl radical in the immune cell membrane, it is regenerated by vitamin C, which is regenerated by glutathione, which is regenerated by glutathione reductase (requiring riboflavin and niacin). The antioxidant chain in immune cells requires all of its members to remain intact during intense immune activity.

Omega-3 resolution requires zinc: The enzymes that convert EPA and DHA to resolvins and protectins include zinc-dependent metalloenzymes. The anti-inflammatory resolution function of omega-3 fatty acids is not solely a function of substrate availability — it depends on the zinc-containing enzymatic machinery that performs the conversion.

The gut microbiome trains the entire orchestra: Every musician in this chapter depends partly on the gut microbiome for its full function: through butyrate-driven Treg development, through IgA production calibrated by microbial signals, through the tryptophan-serotonin-IDO axis that determines the inflammatory character of dendritic cell activation, and through the LPS endotoxemia that results from gut barrier failure and drives the chronic systemic inflammatory activation underlying every autoimmune condition. The immune orchestra cannot be fully tuned without the garden within (Cluster 3).

> *Priya's biological agent suppresses TNF-alpha — one cytokine at the far downstream end of an immune cascade that begins somewhere in the nutritional ecology of her immune system. It does not address the vitamin D deficiency that may be failing to promote regulatory T-cell development. It does not address the omega-3 insufficiency that may be preventing efficient inflammatory resolution. It does not address the gut dysbiosis that removed the primary programmer of the tolerogenic immune circuits that would maintain synovial self-tolerance. The TNF suppressor quiets the alarm. The upstream ecology that produced the alarm remains unmapped.*

VIII. Questions Worth Asking

For a person with an autoimmune condition, recurrent infections that resolve slowly, unusual cancer susceptibility, or a family history of autoimmune disease — the immune nutritional landscape represents an upstream territory that standard rheumatological, oncological, and immunological practice rarely assesses systematically.

Serum 25(OH)D with PTH and magnesium — vitamin D status with its activation context. Serum zinc alongside alkaline phosphatase — zinc with a functional enzyme marker. Serum copper, ceruloplasmin, and RBC copper — copper status with three complementary perspectives. RBC selenium and serum selenoprotein P. Plasma omega-3 index. Anti-TPO alongside selenium status in Hashimoto's. CD4+/CD8+ ratios alongside NK cell activity in individuals with impaired immune surveillance. Stool microbiome assessment for microbiome diversity and butyrate-producing species abundance. These together provide the upstream immune landscape that standard hematology and autoimmune panels cannot capture.

The information in this chapter is educational and does not constitute medical advice. Autoimmune conditions require professional diagnosis and specialist management. Any changes to immunosuppressive therapy must be made in consultation with a treating physician. The author does not offer clinical recommendations for any individual. Selenium supplementation in autoimmune thyroid conditions has documented evidence but requires professional oversight for dose and duration.

IX. Priya's Orchestra, Reconsidered

Eight years. A biological agent that has controlled her symptoms without resolving their cause. A vitamin D that was checked once and found low-normal, with a supplement recommended but not systematically followed. An omega-3 index that has never been measured. A gut microbiome that, after years of processed-food diet and sporadic antibiotic use, has never been assessed or restored. A zinc that has never been measured. A magnesium that has never been measured beyond a serum panel. A complete absence of investigation into the upstream nutritional ecology that educated — or failed to educate — the immune system that is attacking her joints.

The biological agent is doing what it was designed to do. But it was designed to suppress a cytokine. It was not designed to restore the vitamin D-dependent regulatory T-cell development that would maintain immune tolerance. It was not designed to shift the prostaglandin balance from PGE2 amplification to resolvin-mediated resolution. It was not designed to rebuild the gut microbiome whose disruption contributed to the autoimmune permissiveness that preceded her diagnosis by years.

What Priya needed — alongside her pharmacological management, not instead of it — was an investigation of the upstream ecology. The investigation exists. The tools exist. The evidence base exists. The clinical framework that would order the tests, interpret the results, and act on them remains largely absent from the rheumatology clinic where she is managed. The orchestra is playing with eight musicians absent. The conductor is adjusting one section. The concert continues to disappoint.

For the Clinically Curious

Vitamin D and Th17 Suppression — Molecular Mechanism

1,25(OH)2D3 binds to VDR-RXR heterodimers in the regulatory regions of the ROR-gamma-t gene — the master transcription factor for Th17 cell identity. VDR binding suppresses ROR-gamma-t expression, reducing Th17 differentiation and IL-17 production. Simultaneously, VDR signaling upregulates Foxp3 — the Treg master transcription factor — through VDREs in the Foxp3 promoter. The net effect: adequate vitamin D promotes a Treg-dominant regulatory immune state at the expense of Th17 inflammatory activation. This is precisely the balance disrupted in rheumatoid arthritis (elevated Th17, reduced Treg), multiple sclerosis, and inflammatory bowel disease. The VDR-RXR heterodimer also requires retinoid (vitamin A) for full transcriptional activity — connecting vitamin D's immune calibration function to vitamin A status and explaining why combined vitamin A and D insufficiency produces particularly impaired immune regulation.

LFA-1 and Magnesium — The 2022 Cell Paper Mechanism

Gualdoni et al. (Cell, 2022) demonstrated that extracellular magnesium concentrations regulate LFA-1 (lymphocyte function-associated antigen 1, also known as integrin alpha-L beta-2 or CD11a/CD18) conformation on the surface of cytotoxic T-cells and NK cells. LFA-1 transitions between a low-affinity bent conformation and a high-affinity extended conformation; the extended state is required for stable immunological synapse formation with ICAM-1 on target cells. The transition to the high-affinity state requires magnesium binding to the metal ion-dependent adhesion site (MIDAS) of the integrin. In low-magnesium environments (as found in solid tumor microenvironments and in hypomagnesemic individuals), LFA-1 cannot adopt the high-affinity state, the immunological synapse is impaired, and cytotoxic granule delivery is reduced. The paper also demonstrated that magnesium supplementation improved T-cell killing efficiency in both in vitro models and a preclinical mouse model, and suggested that tumor microenvironment magnesium depletion is a mechanism of immune evasion.

Resolvins and Protectins — The Active Resolution Biology

Resolution of inflammation is an active, enzymatically driven process distinct from passive cessation of inflammatory signaling. Resolvin E1 (RvE1, from EPA) and resolvin D1-D6 (from DHA) bind to specific G-protein-coupled receptors on neutrophils (BLT1 for RvE1, GPR32 and ALX/FPR2 for RvD1) and macrophages (ChemR23 for RvE1). Receptor activation halts neutrophil recruitment, promotes macrophage efferocytosis (phagocytosis of apoptotic neutrophils), downregulates NF-κB, and suppresses TNF-alpha production. Protectin D1 (also called neuroprotectin D1 in the CNS) has additional neuroprotective effects via 12-LOX-derived pathway. These resolution mediators are enzymatically synthesized from EPA and DHA, requiring adequate membrane omega-3 fatty acid availability as substrate. The deficit of EPA and DHA in Western populations is therefore a deficit not in anti-inflammatory capacity but in pro-resolution capacity — a mechanistically distinct and clinically important distinction that explains why inflammation that initiates normally in omega-3-depleted individuals may resolve chronically rather than acutely.

Cluster 9

The Methylation Network

How Eight Nutrients Govern Gene Expression, Detoxification, Neurotransmitter Control, and Cardiovascular Risk — and Why the MTHFR Gene Variant Is the Nutritional Insufficiency Medicine Has Relabeled as Genetics

> *"You cannot talk about genes without talking about nutrients. Genes are the instrument. Nutrients play it. The methylation network is where that playing happens — billions of times per day, in every cell, invisibly."*

I. The Gene That Is Not a Sentence

When Catherine received her functional genomics report, it flagged a homozygous MTHFR C677T variant. The accompanying notes explained that this variant reduces the activity of methylenetetrahydrofolate reductase — the enzyme that converts dietary folate to methylfolate, the active form the brain requires for neurotransmitter synthesis, DNA methylation, and the methylation cycle that controls gene expression throughout the body. The report suggested supplementing with methylfolate and methylcobalamin. Catherine's GP had never heard of this and deferred.

The variant is not rare. Approximately ten percent of people of European descent are homozygous for C677T — carrying two copies of the reduced-activity variant. Approximately forty percent carry at least one copy. Catherine is in a significant numerical cohort. The variant does not sentence her to any disease. It narrows her nutritional margin: with adequate methylfolate, active B12, riboflavin (the cofactor for MTHFR itself), B6, betaine, and choline, the methylation cycle functions adequately in most C677T homozygotes. Without this support, it does not.

The variant is not the story. The nutrient status that determines whether the variant is clinically expressed is the story. That status was never assessed. The report named a gene. Nobody asked what the gene needed to perform its function.

II. Meet the Cast

Eight musicians comprise the methylation orchestra. Together they govern the cycle that attaches and removes methyl groups throughout the genome and throughout the body — regulating gene expression, detoxifying neurotransmitters and environmental chemicals, maintaining cardiovascular health through homocysteine management, and providing the biochemical substrate for the synthesis of serotonin, dopamine, melatonin, creatine, phosphatidylcholine, and every other methylated molecule in the body.

- **Folate (as methylfolate)** — Provides the methyl group that regenerates methionine from homocysteine. The MTHFR enzyme produces the active methylfolate form from dietary folate — the step impaired by C677T.
- **Vitamin B12 (methylcobalamin)** — Cofactor for methionine synthase — accepts the methyl group from methylfolate and donates it to homocysteine to regenerate methionine. Without B12, the methyl group transfer stalls and homocysteine accumulates regardless of folate status.
- **Vitamin B6 (pyridoxal-5-phosphate)** — Required for the transsulfuration pathway — the alternative route by which excess homocysteine is converted to cysteine rather than recycled to methionine. Also required for serine hydroxymethyltransferase, which feeds one-carbon units into the folate cycle.
- **Riboflavin (B2)** — Cofactor for MTHFR itself. MTHFR activity is reduced not only by genetic variants but by riboflavin insufficiency — which impairs even normal MTHFR function. Riboflavin supplementation has been shown in clinical trials to significantly reduce homocysteine specifically in C677T homozygotes.
- **Choline** — Precursor to betaine (trimethylglycine), the methyl donor in the betaine-homocysteine methyltransferase (BHMT) pathway — the alternative,

folate-independent route for homocysteine remethylation. Provides the methylation backup when the folate-B12 route is impaired.

- **Betaine (trimethylglycine)** — The direct methyl donor in the BHMT pathway. Can reduce homocysteine independently of MTHFR, folate, and B12, making it a nutritionally accessible pathway particularly valuable for those with MTHFR variants or B12 insufficiency.
- **Zinc** — Required for DNA methyltransferases — the enzymes that attach methyl groups to cytosine residues in DNA to regulate gene expression. Zinc deficiency impairs epigenetic DNA methylation patterns independent of the folate-B12 cycle.
- **Magnesium** — Cofactor for methionine adenosyltransferase (MAT) — the enzyme that converts methionine to SAMe using ATP. Also required for multiple other ATP-dependent methylation cycle steps. As with virtually every enzymatic process in the body, magnesium is the activation key.

These eight musicians govern the methylation cycle — the body's universal methyl group delivery system. Their collective sufficiency determines whether DNA is correctly silenced and expressed, whether neurotransmitters are properly inactivated, whether homocysteine accumulates or is cleared, and whether the body can synthesize the billions of methylated molecules it requires each day for normal function.

III. The Methylation Cycle — A Map for the General Reader

Methylation is the attachment of a methyl group — one carbon atom bonded to three hydrogen atoms (CH3) — to another molecule. This small chemical addition changes the molecule's properties profoundly: silencing a gene when the methyl group attaches to DNA, deactivating a neurotransmitter when it attaches to dopamine or adrenaline, tagging a toxic compound for liver excretion, or providing the building block for creatine, carnitine, or phosphatidylcholine.

The cycle that supplies these methyl groups works as follows. Dietary methionine — an essential amino acid from protein — is converted to SAMe (S-adenosylmethionine) by methionine adenosyltransferase, using ATP as a cofactor (which requires magnesium). SAMe is the universal methyl donor — it donates its methyl group to whatever target requires it, becoming SAH (S-adenosylhomocysteine) and then homocysteine in the process. Homocysteine sits at a metabolic crossroads: it can be remethylated back to methionine (via the folate-B12 route, driven by methylfolate donating its methyl group through methionine synthase, or via the choline-betaine route through BHMT), or it can be directed into the transsulfuration pathway (via B6-dependent cystathionine beta-synthase) to produce cysteine — which flows on to glutathione production, taurine synthesis, and sulfate conjugation for detoxification.

Every rotation of this cycle consumes methyl groups, depends on the eight nutrients above, and generates either a remethylated methionine (recycling the cycle) or a cysteine (feeding antioxidant and detoxification pathways). The cycle runs billions of times per day in every cell of the body. Its insufficiency — whether from MTHFR variants, B12 depletion, folate inadequacy, or riboflavin deficiency — produces homocysteine accumulation, reduced SAMe availability, and impaired DNA methylation that have consequences for cardiovascular health, neurological function, gene expression, and detoxification capacity simultaneously.

Homocysteine — The Cardiovascular Marker Medicine Ignores

When the methylation cycle is insufficient — from any combination of impaired MTHFR activity, B12 depletion, folate inadequacy, or riboflavin deficiency — homocysteine accumulates in the blood. Elevated homocysteine is an independent risk factor for cardiovascular disease, stroke, venous thromboembolism, depression, cognitive decline, and dementia. The cardiovascular risk mechanism is endothelial dysfunction: homocysteine directly damages arterial endothelial cells, impairs nitric oxide production, generates reactive oxygen species that oxidize LDL, promotes platelet aggregation, and activates the coagulation cascade.

The Homocysteine Studies Collaboration meta-analysis — pooling data from over 30 prospective studies — found that a 3 micromol/L lower homocysteine was associated with an approximately eleven percent lower coronary heart disease risk and a nineteen percent lower stroke risk. These associations are consistent, replicated, and biologically explained by the endothelial mechanism. The B vitamin intervention that lowers homocysteine — folate, B12, B6 — is inexpensive, safe, and effective. Homocysteine testing costs a few dollars. It is not on the routine cardiovascular panel in most clinical settings, because it leads to a nutritional intervention rather than a pharmaceutical one.

In pregnancy, homocysteine above seven micromol/L is associated with increased neural tube defect risk — explaining why periconceptional folate supplementation is one of the most unambiguous public health interventions in nutritional medicine. The same biochemistry that produces the neural tube risk — impaired methylation-dependent fetal neural development — produces cardiovascular and neurological risk throughout adult life. The folate-pregnancy relationship is established and acted upon. The folate-adult cardiovascular and neurological relationship is documented and largely ignored.

IV. SAMe — The Methyl Donor the Brain Needs

SAMe (S-adenosylmethionine) is the biochemical endpoint of the methylation cycle — the molecule that actually donates methyl groups to the hundreds of different methylation reactions in the body. Its targets include: DNA cytosine residues (gene silencing), RNA (post-transcriptional modification), histones (chromatin structure regulation), phosphatidylcholine (neuronal membrane building), creatine (muscle energy buffer), carnitine (fatty acid transport), melatonin (from serotonin via N-acetylation and methylation), and the inactivation of dopamine, noradrenaline, and adrenaline by catechol-O-methyltransferase (COMT).

SAMe concentrations in the brain correlate directly with mood. SAMe supplementation has been studied as an antidepressant in multiple randomized controlled trials, with results demonstrating efficacy comparable to tricyclic antidepressants in mild to moderate depression and significant augmentation of SSRI response in partial responders. Its mechanism is distinct from SSRIs: SAMe supports the methylation of neurotransmitter inactivation enzymes (ensuring appropriate turnover), the production of phosphatidylcholine for neuronal membrane integrity, and the synthesis of creatine that buffers neuronal energy. In individuals with impaired methylation cycles — from MTHFR variants, B12 insufficiency, or folate depletion — SAMe production is reduced at baseline, creating a substrate deficit that pharmacological antidepressants cannot address because they act downstream of the synthesis pathway they depend on.

V. The Transsulfuration Pathway — Where Methylation Meets Antioxidant Defense

When homocysteine is not remethylated to methionine, it can be diverted into the transsulfuration pathway: cystathionine beta-synthase (requiring B6) converts homocysteine and serine to cystathionine, which gamma-cystathionase (also B6-dependent) then converts to cysteine. Cysteine is the rate-limiting precursor for glutathione synthesis — directly connecting the methylation network to the antioxidant network of Cluster 4.

This connection has a profound clinical implication. Individuals with impaired methylation cycles — whether from MTHFR variants, B12 deficiency, or folate depletion — may have reduced glutathione production capacity even when their dietary glycine and cysteine intakes are adequate, because the transsulfuration pathway that supplies cysteine depends on the homocysteine that the methylation cycle generates. An impaired methylation cycle simultaneously elevates homocysteine (cardiovascular risk) and reduces cysteine flow into glutathione (antioxidant insufficiency) — two distinct harms from a single upstream cause.

Understanding this connection helps explain a clinical pattern seen in many MTHFR variant carriers: concurrent elevation of plasma homocysteine alongside markers of increased oxidative stress, with both being downstream consequences of the same methylation impairment. Addressing the methylation network — with methylfolate, B12, riboflavin, B6, betaine — resolves both consequences simultaneously through a single upstream intervention.

VI. Epigenetics — The Methylation Network's Most Consequential Role

Gene expression is not fixed. It is regulated continuously by the availability of methyl groups from SAMe, which silence gene promoters through DNA methyltransferase-mediated methylation of cytosine residues adjacent to guanine (CpG sites). Adequate SAMe production — dependent on the full methylation network —

maintains the epigenetic regulation patterns that determine which genes are expressed in which tissues, when, and at what levels. Insufficient SAMe production leads to hypomethylation of gene promoters that should be silenced — including proto-oncogenes and pro-inflammatory genes — and potentially altered expression of genes governing cellular differentiation, growth control, and immune function.

The epigenetic consequences of methylation impairment are long-term and cumulative. They are not detectable on any standard blood panel and do not announce themselves as a diagnosable condition until the epigenetic drift has produced sufficient downstream pathology to cross a clinical threshold. They represent, in Bruce Ames's triage framework, the long-term harms that a chronically insufficient methylation network accumulates silently while prioritizing the most immediate functions — neurotransmitter synthesis, creatine production, energy metabolism — that maintain day-to-day function.

The reversibility of DNA methylation patterns — epigenetic marks can be added and removed throughout life — means that correcting methylation insufficiency is not a futile exercise for adults with pre-existing epigenetic drift. The marks can be reset. The genes can be re-silenced. The window for intervention is open at any age, even if the most consequential period for establishing methylation patterns is early development.

VII. The Web of Dependencies

Folate requires riboflavin: MTHFR — the enzyme that converts dietary folate to active methylfolate — requires riboflavin (FAD) as its cofactor. Riboflavin deficiency reduces MTHFR activity as effectively as some genetic variants. The clinical expression of C677T is more severe in riboflavin-insufficient individuals. Riboflavin supplementation in C677T homozygotes has been shown to reduce homocysteine significantly, independent of folate and B12 status.

B12 requires folate — and the reverse: Methionine synthase requires both methylfolate (the methyl donor) and methylcobalamin (the B12 form that accepts and transfers the methyl group) to function. Either alone is insufficient. The classical clinical trap: high-dose folic acid supplementation without B12 may mask the hematological signs of B12 deficiency while neurological demyelination continues — because the hematological effect requires folate, but the neurological effect requires both.

Choline provides the bypass: The BHMT pathway — using betaine from choline as a methyl donor — bypasses the MTHFR-dependent step entirely. Individuals with impaired folate methylation who have adequate choline and betaine may compensate partially through this pathway. This explains why dietary choline adequacy modifies the clinical severity of MTHFR variants — a nutritional modifier of genetic risk that is rarely assessed.

Methylation connects to detoxification: COMT-mediated methylation of estrogens and catecholamines uses SAMe, drawing from the same methyl donor pool that serves DNA methylation and neurotransmitter regulation. High environmental toxin loads or high hormone turnover increases SAMe demand for detoxification, potentially compromising methylation availability for neurological and epigenetic functions — connecting Clusters 9 and 10 at their shared methyl group currency.

Transsulfuration connects to glutathione: As described above, the methylation cycle is the upstream source of cysteine for glutathione synthesis. Impaired methylation impairs antioxidant defense through this cysteine connection — linking Clusters 9 and 4 through a shared biochemical intermediate.

> *Catherine's MTHFR C677T variant does not determine her fate. It narrows her nutritional margin — her requirement for methylfolate, B12, riboflavin, and choline is higher than average, and the consequences of failing to meet that requirement are more severe. Given the nutrients the gene needs to function, the variant is a footnote. Given the typical Western diet's provision of those nutrients, it becomes a bottleneck with cascading consequences. The gene is not the story. The nutrient status that determines its expression is the story. That status was never assessed. The report named the gene and stopped.*

VIII. Questions Worth Asking

For a person with unexplained cardiovascular risk, treatment-resistant depression, recurrent pregnancy loss, neural tube defect history, cognitive decline, persistent fatigue, or a known MTHFR variant — the methylation network is an upstream territory whose assessment is both accessible and highly actionable.

Fasting plasma total homocysteine — the primary functional marker of methylation cycle sufficiency. RBC folate alongside plasma folate — the tissue-level store alongside the recent intake picture. Serum B12 alongside plasma methylmalonic acid — serum B12 as a gross screen, MMA as the functional marker that reveals cellular B12 insufficiency when serum appears normal. Plasma pyridoxal-5-phosphate for active B6 status. Plasma betaine and choline for the backup methylation pathway substrate. MTHFR C677T and A1298C genotyping for variant status that refines interpretation of all other measures. Plasma riboflavin or RBC glutathione reductase activation coefficient for riboflavin functional status. Serum zinc alongside alkaline phosphatase for zinc's epigenetic methylation role.

The information in this chapter is educational and does not constitute clinical advice. The management of MTHFR variants, elevated homocysteine, and methylation-related conditions requires individualized professional assessment. High-dose folate supplementation during pregnancy requires medical guidance. The author does not offer clinical recommendations for any individual. MTHFR testing and interpretation should be discussed with a qualified healthcare professional familiar with nutritional genomics.

IX. Catherine's Orchestra, Reconsidered

Catherine's MTHFR C677T report named a gene. Nobody measured what the gene needed. Her riboflavin status — the cofactor for the very enzyme whose gene was reported as reduced-function — has never been assessed. Her plasma homocysteine has never been measured. Her active B12 status has never been confirmed with methylmalonic acid. Her choline intake — the backup pathway that could compensate for impaired MTHFR function — has never been discussed. Her betaine status has never been measured.

What Catherine has is a narrower nutritional margin than most. She requires more methylfolate, more B12, more riboflavin, and more choline to achieve the same methylation cycle efficiency that most people achieve on a standard diet. With adequate nutritional support, her variant is a minor footnote — the kind of genetic variation that a well-nourished body handles without producing symptoms. Without that support, it becomes the upstream explanation for her elevated cardiovascular risk, her treatment-resistant mood instability, and her impaired DNA methylation — consequences that will be treated downstream with statins, antidepressants, and ever more sophisticated management of diseases whose nutritional root has never been addressed.

The report told Catherine she had a gene variant. What it should have told her is that she has a specific nutritional requirement — a nutritional margin that the variant has narrowed, and that the right combination of methylfolate, B12, riboflavin, B6, and choline can restore. The distinction between those two framings is the distinction between a genetic sentence and a nutritional strategy. One forecloses. The other opens.

For the Clinically Curious

MTHFR C677T — Enzyme Biochemistry and Population Frequency

MTHFR (methylenetetrahydrofolate reductase) catalyzes the reduction of 5,10-methylenetetrahydrofolate to 5-methyltetrahydrofolate (methylfolate), using NADPH and FAD as cofactors. The C677T variant (rs1801133) encodes an Ala→Val substitution at position 222 that reduces enzyme thermostability and catalytic efficiency. Heterozygotes show approximately 35% reduced activity; homozygotes approximately 65% reduced activity relative to wild-type. The A1298C variant (rs1801131) reduces activity approximately 20% in heterozygotes. Compound heterozygosity (one C677T + one A1298C) produces intermediate impairment. Population frequencies of C677T homozygosity: ~10% European, ~8% South Asian, ~20-25% Southern European and Mexican, ~2-5% sub-Saharan African. Clinical expression varies dramatically with riboflavin, folate, and B12 status — populations with high riboflavin intakes (from whole grains or supplementation) show minimal homocysteine elevation even in C677T homozygotes, confirming the nutritional modifiability of this genetic risk.

SAMe in Depression — The Evidence Base

SAMe has been studied as an antidepressant since the 1970s. A 2004 meta-analysis (Mischoulon and Fava) found SAMe superior to placebo and comparable to tricyclic antidepressants in mild to moderate depression. A landmark randomized trial (Papakostas et al., American Journal of Psychiatry, 2010) found that SAMe (800 mg twice daily) as an adjunct to SSRIs significantly improved treatment response rates (36% vs 18%

response, 26% vs 12% remission, p<0.05) in SSRI-partial-responders over 6 weeks. A 2014 systematic review and meta-analysis confirmed SAMe's antidepressant efficacy across multiple study designs. The mechanism — supporting methylation of neurotransmitter synthesis enzymes, providing substrate for phosphatidylcholine in neuronal membranes, and directly influencing catecholamine turnover through COMT methylation — is distinct from SSRI mechanisms and provides a non-competitive adjunct rationale. SAMe's evidence base, by any objective methodological standard, would support clinical recommendation in psychiatry — if it were a patentable pharmaceutical rather than a nutritional compound.

Homocysteine Reduction with B Vitamins — Stroke Prevention Evidence

The HOPE-2 trial (NEJM, 2006) demonstrated that combined B6, B12, and folate supplementation significantly reduced homocysteine by approximately 2.4 micromol/L over 5 years but did not significantly reduce cardiovascular events in the overall study population of 5,522 vascular disease patients. However, subsequent analysis and the China Stroke Primary Prevention Trial (CSPPT, JAMA, 2015) demonstrated significant stroke reduction (21%) with folic acid supplementation in 20,702 hypertensive adults without prior stroke or cardiovascular disease, particularly in individuals with low baseline folate. The divergence between HOPE-2 (secondary prevention, no benefit) and CSPPT (primary prevention, significant benefit) is consistent with the hypothesis that homocysteine-mediated vascular damage is most effectively prevented before established disease is present — reinforcing the case for upstream assessment and intervention rather than downstream addition to existing cardiovascular management.

Epigenetic Clock and Methylation — The Aging Connection

The Horvath epigenetic clock — a DNA methylation-based biological age estimator derived from CpG methylation patterns at 353 sites — has become one of the most validated biomarkers of biological aging. Accelerated epigenetic aging (biological age exceeding chronological age by the clock) is associated with increased all-cause mortality, cancer risk, and neurodegeneration, independent of other risk factors. Methylation sufficiency — adequate SAMe production from the folate-B12-betaine network — is required to maintain the CpG methylation patterns that the clock uses as age markers. Studies have found that B12 deficiency, elevated homocysteine, and reduced dietary folate are associated with accelerated epigenetic clock aging. Conversely, supplementation with methylation network nutrients has shown trends toward deceleration of epigenetic clock aging in small intervention studies. The methylation network's influence on biological aging — through its epigenetic maintenance function — represents one of the most consequential and least discussed dimensions of nutritional geroscience.

Cluster 10

The Detoxification Network

How the Body Eliminates What It Cannot Use — and Why Chronic Illness, Chemical Sensitivity, and Hormonal Imbalance Are Often Detoxification Stories Medicine Has Never Read

"The body is not passive in the face of the modern chemical world. It was built to detoxify. What it was not built for is a world that delivers toxins faster than the nutrients required to eliminate them can keep pace."

I. The Body's Processing Plant

Margaret takes five medications. She lives in a suburban home with off-gassing carpets and synthetic cleaning products. She drinks water from aged pipes. She eats conventionally grown produce sprayed with pesticide residues. She breathes air that contains vehicle exhaust, industrial particulates, and volatile organic compounds. She has been under chronic psychological stress for a decade, producing a continuous stream of cortisol metabolites that her liver must process and excrete. And nobody —

in all the years she has been seen by physicians — has ever asked how well her body is handling this load.

The liver processes every molecule that enters the bloodstream from the gut, the lungs, the skin, or the bloodstream itself. It is the body's chemical processing plant — the site where medications are metabolized, where environmental toxins are neutralized, where hormones are inactivated after their signaling work is done, where alcohol is converted to acetaldehyde and then to acetate, and where the thousands of endogenous and exogenous chemical species that enter the body each day are modified for excretion. This processing is not a single reaction. It is a two-phase system, and both phases depend critically on nutritional cofactors that modern diets frequently fail to provide at adequate levels.

II. Meet the Cast

The detoxification network involves nutrients across several clusters — it is the most cross-referencing section of the book. But the core musicians are:

- **Glutathione** — The master phase II conjugator — the molecule that attaches to activated toxins to make them water-soluble for urinary or biliary excretion. The liver's primary chemical defense.
- **Glycine** — Phase II conjugation amino acid — conjugates with benzoic acid derivatives, bile acids, and other

compounds for excretion. Also required for glutathione synthesis.

- **Taurine** — Phase II conjugator for bile acids and certain drugs. Also a neuroprotective amino acid and cellular osmoregulator.
- **N-acetylcysteine (NAC)** — Cysteine donor for glutathione synthesis. The primary clinical intervention for glutathione depletion — used in acetaminophen overdose precisely because it restores liver glutathione.
- **Sulfur (methionine and cysteine)** — Source of the sulfate groups used in sulfation — one of the most important phase II conjugation reactions for steroid hormones, neurotransmitters, and phenolic compounds.
- **Molybdenum** — Cofactor for sulfite oxidase and xanthine oxidase; completes the sulfur-processing pathway that Phase II conjugation depends on.
- **B vitamins (B2, B3, B6, B12, folate)** — Essential cofactors for phase I cytochrome P450 enzymes and for the methylation reactions that constitute a major phase II pathway.
- **Magnesium** — Required for phase I enzyme activity and for the ATP-dependent phase II conjugation reactions.
- **Zinc and selenium** — Cofactors for superoxide dismutase and glutathione peroxidase — the antioxidant enzymes that neutralize the reactive intermediates generated by phase I processing.

The detoxification network is uniquely dependent on nutrients from multiple other clusters — it sits downstream of energy production, methylation, antioxidant defense, and amino acid supply simultaneously. It is, in this sense, the cluster that shows most clearly what happens when the whole orchestra is short-staffed.

III. Phase I and Phase II — The Two-Stage System

Phase I — Activation, Not Elimination

Phase I detoxification is performed by the cytochrome P450 enzyme family — a group of heme-containing enzymes located primarily in the liver's endoplasmic reticulum. Phase I reactions modify toxins through oxidation, reduction, and hydrolysis reactions, making them more chemically reactive — not less. This is counterintuitive but essential: most lipid-soluble toxins cannot be directly excreted because they would be reabsorbed in the kidney tubules before reaching the urine. They must first be chemically modified in a way that allows phase II conjugation to attach a water-soluble group that enables excretion.

The problem is that phase I reactions generate reactive intermediates — often more chemically reactive and potentially more toxic than the original compound. These intermediates cause oxidative stress if not immediately captured and conjugated by phase II enzymes. When phase I is active but phase II is overwhelmed or nutrient-depleted, reactive intermediates accumulate, damage cellular proteins and DNA, and produce the oxidative stress characteristic of toxin overload. This is why stimulating detoxification — through sauna, fasting, or certain supplements — without supporting the complete two-phase system can paradoxically worsen outcomes. Phase I without phase II creates more damage, not less.

Phase I enzymes require: riboflavin (FAD), niacin (NADP+), magnesium, iron (in the heme group), and adequate protein for enzyme synthesis. Importantly, phase I activity is upregulated by many medications — including the five medications Margaret takes — meaning that her pharmacological management has increased the demand on a liver processing system whose nutritional support has never been assessed.

Phase II — Conjugation and Excretion

Phase II detoxification attaches water-soluble groups to the reactive phase I intermediates, producing conjugates that can be excreted in urine or bile. The major phase II pathways are:

Glutathione conjugation: *Glutathione S-transferases attach glutathione to reactive electrophiles — including activated environmental toxins, activated drug metabolites, and lipid peroxidation products. This is the highest-capacity phase II pathway and the one most rapidly overwhelmed in toxin overload. Glutathione synthesis requires glycine, cysteine, and glutamate, with adequate B6, magnesium, and selenium for the enzyme systems that regenerate and deploy it.*

Methylation: *Catechol-O-methyltransferase (COMT) and other methyltransferases inactivate catecholamines (dopamine, adrenaline, noradrenaline), estrogens, and certain drugs by attaching methyl groups. This directly connects the methylation network (Cluster 9) to detoxification — SAMe provides the methyl group, folate and B12 regenerate SAMe, and COMT activity determines the rate at which estrogens and catecholamines are cleared.*

Sulfation: *Sulfotransferases attach sulfate groups to steroid hormones, thyroid hormone, and phenolic compounds. Sulfate is derived from cysteine and methionine via the transsulfuration pathway — connecting sulfur amino acid adequacy directly to hormone clearance. Estrogen sulfation is the primary route by which the liver inactivates estrogens for excretion; insufficient sulfation capacity contributes to estrogen dominance.*

Glucuronidation: *UDP-glucuronosyltransferases attach glucuronic acid to hormones, drugs, and bilirubin, producing glucuronide conjugates excreted in bile. This pathway requires UDP-glucuronic acid derived from glucose metabolism and is one of the primary routes for bilirubin clearance, estrogen conjugation, and drug metabolism.*

Amino acid conjugation: *Glycine, taurine, and glutamine conjugate with certain acids and drugs to form water-soluble derivatives. Glycine conjugates with benzoic acid (a common food preservative) and bile acids; taurine conjugates with bile acids and* *certain drugs. Glycine and taurine depletion directly impairs this pathway.*

Molybdenum is the mineral that closes the sulfur loop. As the cofactor for sulfite oxidase, it converts the sulfite generated when sulfur-containing amino acids are broken down into harmless sulfate — the same sulfate the body then draws on for Phase II sulfation. Without adequate molybdenum, sulfite accumulates rather than converting, and the sulfate supply that sulfation conjugation depends on runs short. Molybdenum is also the cofactor for xanthine oxidase and aldehyde oxidase, two further clearance enzymes. It is needed only in trace amounts and is rarely measured, but a diet low in legumes, whole grains, and leafy greens — its principal sources — can leave this final step of the sulfur pathway under-supplied.

IV. The Estrogen-Detoxification Connection

Estrogen metabolism is one of the most clinically important applications of the detoxification framework. The liver processes estrogen through a sequence of phase I hydroxylation reactions that can produce protective metabolites (2-hydroxyoestrone, 2-methoxyoestrone) or proliferative metabolites (16-alpha-hydroxyoestrone, 4-hydroxyoestrone) depending on which cytochrome P450 enzymes are most active. Phase II then inactivates all of these metabolites through methylation (COMT), sulfation, and glucuronidation for excretion.

The balance between protective and proliferative estrogen metabolites is directly affected by nutritional status. Indole-3-carbinol (I3C) and diindolylmethane (DIM) — compounds derived from cruciferous vegetables — shift phase I estrogen metabolism toward the 2-hydroxylation pathway, producing less proliferative metabolites. Adequate COMT function (requiring magnesium and SAMe) ensures methylation of 2-hydroxyoestrone to the fully inactivated 2-methoxyoestrone. Adequate sulfation (requiring cysteine, methionine, and molybdenum) further clears estrogen conjugates for biliary excretion. Fiber and a healthy microbiome prevent beta-glucuronidase — a bacterial enzyme that uncouples glucuronide conjugates in the colon — from recycling cleared estrogens back into the circulation.

When any of these steps is impaired — through nutritional insufficiency, gut dysbiosis producing high beta-glucuronidase activity, or methylation pathway impairment from MTHFR variants — estrogen exposure is extended and the balance between metabolite types shifts. The clinical consequences are felt in conditions characterized by excess or imbalanced estrogen activity: endometriosis, fibroids, premenstrual syndrome, and breast cancer risk. These conditions are almost exclusively managed at their symptomatic endpoints. The upstream detoxification ecology — assessable with urinary estrogen metabolite testing — is rarely the focus of clinical investigation.

V. The Heavy Metal Connection

The detoxification network is the body's primary defense against heavy metal accumulation. Lead, mercury, arsenic, cadmium, and aluminum — all present in the modern environment through food, water, amalgam dental fillings, industrial exposure, and contaminated soil — are processed through phase II conjugation pathways that depend on glutathione, cysteine, and the sulfur-containing amino acids. Alpha-lipoic acid chelates mercury and arsenic. Selenium forms insoluble selenides with mercury, reducing its bioavailability. Zinc competes with cadmium for absorption.

When the detoxification network is nutritionally depleted — when glutathione is low, when cysteine and glycine are insufficient, when selenium is marginal — the body's capacity to sequester and excrete heavy metals is reduced. Metals accumulate in tissues: lead in bone, mercury in neuronal myelin and kidney tubules, cadmium in the kidney cortex, arsenic in hair and nails. Accumulated metals then impair the very enzyme systems that would otherwise process them — creating a self-reinforcing cycle of toxic burden and nutritional depletion that standard medicine addresses neither upstream (nutritional support) nor downstream (metal elimination) except in cases of frank poisoning.

VI. The Web of Dependencies

Phase I generates what phase II must eliminate: The single most important clinical principle of detoxification biochemistry. Stimulating phase I without supporting phase II creates reactive intermediates that damage cells. The nutritional support for both phases must be concurrent.

Glutathione connects all clusters: Glutathione requires glycine and cysteine (amino acid cluster), is regenerated by riboflavin and niacin (energy cluster), protects against phase I oxidative stress (antioxidant cluster), and is the primary conjugator for environmental toxins (detoxification cluster). It is the single most cross-referenced molecule in the book.

Methylation is shared with cluster 9: COMT-mediated methylation of estrogens and catecholamines consumes SAMe — the same methyl donor that the methylation network uses for DNA methylation, neurotransmitter regulation, and myelin maintenance. A person with high toxin load and high hormone turnover has elevated SAMe demand, which may compromise methylation availability for neurological and epigenetic functions.

> *The body was not built for the modern chemical world. It was built for the chemical world of 50,000 years ago — where environmental toxin exposure was episodic, the nutrient supply was abundant, and the detoxification network was adequately resourced. In the modern world, the toxin load is continuous, the*

> *nutrient supply is marginal, and the processing plant is running at capacity on depleted fuel. The illness that results is not a disease. It is an engineering problem — and it has a nutritional solution.*

VII. Questions Worth Asking

For a person with chemical sensitivity, unexplained fatigue, hormonal imbalance, persistent skin conditions, poor drug tolerance (medications either barely work or produce side effects at standard doses), or a significant environmental exposure history — the detoxification network represents upstream territory worth exploring.

Urinary organic acids assess phase I and phase II intermediates and can identify bottlenecks in specific pathways. Urinary estrogen metabolite testing (DUTCH test or equivalent) reveals the hydroxylation balance and the efficiency of downstream inactivation. Glutathione (RBC), cysteine, glycine, and taurine levels can be measured in plasma. Genetic testing for CYP450 polymorphisms (the major phase I enzymes) and COMT is commercially available. Heavy metal testing — hair mineral analysis for chronic exposure, urine challenge testing for mobilizable stores, or blood testing for acute exposure — rounds out the picture.

The information in this chapter is educational and does not constitute medical advice. Detoxification support protocols require individualized clinical assessment. Heavy metal testing and intervention should be supervised by a qualified healthcare professional. The author does not offer clinical recommendations for any individual.

For the Clinically Curious

Cytochrome P450 Enzymes — Genetic Variation and Clinical Significance

The CYP450 superfamily comprises more than 50 enzymes in humans, of which CYP1A2, CYP2C9, CYP2C19, CYP2D6, and CYP3A4/5 are responsible for the metabolism of the majority of clinically used drugs. Each gene has common variants that produce poor metaboliser (PM), intermediate metaboliser (IM), extensive metaboliser (EM), and ultra-rapid metaboliser (UM) phenotypes. CYP2D6 PMs — approximately 7–10% of European populations — cannot effectively metabolize codeine to morphine (reducing analgesic effect) or tamoxifen to endoxifen (reducing anti-cancer efficacy), while UMs metabolize these drugs so rapidly that standard doses are ineffective. CYP2C19 PMs cannot activate clopidogrel (a common antiplatelet drug), significantly increasing cardiovascular event risk post-stenting. Pharmacogenomic testing for CYP450 variants is commercially available and increasingly used in clinical practice — but the nutritional status that modulates CYP450 enzyme activity (riboflavin, niacin, magnesium, iron) is never concurrently assessed.

Beta-Glucuronidase and Estrogen Recycling

Beta-glucuronidase is produced by gut bacteria including Bacteroides, Clostridium, and E. coli species. It cleaves glucuronide conjugates in the colon, releasing free estrogens from their conjugated form — allowing them to be reabsorbed rather than excreted. High beta-glucuronidase activity (measurable in stool analysis) effectively recirculates estrogens that the liver has conjugated for excretion, prolonging estrogen exposure and contributing to estrogen dominance. Dietary fiber, calcium D-glucarate (a food compound in cruciferous vegetables and citrus), and a diverse microbiome all reduce beta-glucuronidase activity. This mechanism is one of the most clinically important connections between gut microbiome health and hormonal balance, and it is virtually absent from conventional gynecological or oncological clinical discussion.

Glutathione S-Transferase Polymorphisms — GSTM1 and GSTT1 Null Genotypes

GSTM1 and GSTT1 null polymorphisms — homozygous deletions of glutathione S-transferase genes — produce complete absence of the corresponding enzymes. GSTM1 null affects approximately 50% of European populations; GSTT1 null affects approximately 20%. Individuals with null genotypes in either gene have reduced glutathione conjugation capacity for their respective substrates — including carcinogens, heavy metals, and oxidative stress products. GSTM1 and GSTT1 null genotypes are associated with increased cancer risk across multiple tumor sites, consistent with reduced detoxification capacity. The clinical significance is nutritionally modifiable: glutathione precursor sufficiency (NAC, glycine) is more critical in null genotype carriers because their reduced enzyme capacity amplifies the impact of any substrate-level limitation.

Cluster 11

The Amino Acid Foundation

How Protein's Building Blocks Govern Muscle, Neurotransmitters, Immune Defense, and the Entire Fabric of the Body — and Why the Source and Completeness of Protein Is Medicine's Most Overlooked Macronutrient Story

"We are not what we eat. We are what we absorb, and what we build from what we absorb. Protein is not fuel. It is the raw material for everything else in this book."

I. The Forgotten Macronutrient

Nutrition science has spent decades debating fat and carbohydrates. The glycemic index, saturated fat, seed oils, ketosis, low-fat diets, Mediterranean diets — the macronutrient conversation has been almost entirely about fat and carbohydrate. Protein has been reduced to a simple question — how much? — that misses the more important questions: which amino acids, from which sources, and whether the full complement of essential and conditionally essential amino acids is actually reaching the cells that need them.

The body cannot store amino acids in the way it stores fat and glycogen. The amino acid pool — the free amino acids available in blood and tissues — turns over continuously, and any amino acid that is consistently undersupplied creates a bottleneck in every synthesis pathway that requires it. The body manages these bottlenecks through triage — prioritizing the most immediately critical functions while downregulating the less urgent ones. Muscle is sacrificed before organ function. Glutathione synthesis is downregulated before immunoglobulin production. Collagen synthesis slows before enzyme production. The triage is silent and systematic, and its consequences accumulate over years before they are visible in any standard blood panel.

II. Meet the Cast

Fourteen amino acids deserve individual attention in this chapter — the nine essential amino acids that the body cannot synthesize at all, plus five conditionally essential ones whose deficiency is so consequential and so prevalent in modern populations that they function as de facto essential nutrients.

- **Leucine** — The primary trigger for muscle protein synthesis through mTOR signaling. Without adequate leucine, dietary protein does not stimulate anabolism regardless of total protein intake.

- **Lysine** — Required for carnitine synthesis, collagen hydroxylation, and immune peptide synthesis. Depleted by high-cereal diets. The limiting amino acid in most plant-based proteins.
- **Methionine** — The only sulfur-containing essential amino acid. Initiates every protein synthesis event (as the start codon). Precursor to SAMe, cysteine, and taurine.
- **Tryptophan** — Sole precursor of serotonin and melatonin. Also the primary substrate for NAD+ synthesis via the kynurenine pathway — connecting it to the energy network.
- **Threonine** — Rate-limiting amino acid for gut mucin synthesis. Required for glycine and serine production.
- **Isoleucine** — One of the three branched-chain amino acids. Supports skeletal muscle glucose uptake during exercise, contributes to muscle protein synthesis alongside leucine, and plays a role in immune defense through production of antimicrobial peptides in the gut epithelium.
- **Valine** — The third branched-chain amino acid. Provides energy substrate for skeletal muscle during exercise and illness, supports tissue repair and nitrogen balance, and is metabolized directly in muscle rather than in the liver — making the BCAAs uniquely available as fast-acting fuel during physical stress.
- **Phenylalanine** — Precursor to tyrosine, and through tyrosine, to dopamine, noradrenaline, adrenaline, thyroid hormone, and melanin. Connects directly to Clusters 6 and 7.
- **Histidine** — Required for hemoglobin production and histamine synthesis. The imidazole ring of histidine is

required for the catalytic activity of multiple metalloenzymes.

- **Glycine (conditionally essential)** — The most underconsumed structural amino acid. Rate-limiting for collagen synthesis, glutathione production, and bile acid conjugation. Synthesized endogenously but far below requirement.
- **Glutamine (conditionally essential)** — Primary fuel for enterocytes and rapidly dividing immune cells. Becomes essential during illness, injury, and intensive exercise.
- **Cysteine (conditionally essential)** — Rate-limiting precursor for glutathione. Produced from methionine via the transsulfuration pathway but frequently insufficient in the modern diet and under oxidative stress.
- **Taurine (conditionally essential)** — Synthesized from cysteine but often insufficient. Required for bile acid conjugation, neurological function, cardiovascular regulation, and osmoregulation.
- **Arginine (conditionally essential)** — Substrate for nitric oxide synthesis and the urea cycle's ammonia-clearing step. Endogenous synthesis is normally adequate but is outstripped during illness, trauma, and cardiovascular strain — precisely when its role in vascular tone matters most.

III. The Protein Quality Problem

Essential vs. Complete

Nine amino acids cannot be synthesized by the human body at all — they must come from food. A protein source that contains all nine in proportions that meet human requirements is called complete. Animal proteins — meat, fish, eggs, dairy — are complete. Most plant proteins are not, being deficient in one or more essential amino acids. Wheat is low in lysine. Rice is low in lysine and threonine. Legumes are low in methionine and cysteine. Corn is low in lysine and tryptophan.

For most of human history, dietary protein came predominantly from animal sources — meat, fish, eggs, and dairy — that provided complete amino acid profiles. The shift toward plant-predominant diets, however well-motivated by environmental and health considerations, creates a systematic risk of amino acid insufficiency unless specific complementation strategies are employed. A person eating predominantly rice and beans can achieve adequate protein intake in grams while remaining deficient in specific essential amino acids whose dietary sources they are not consuming.

The concept of protein complementation — eating different plant proteins together to ensure a complete essential amino acid profile — is sound in theory but requires knowledge and intentionality that most people do not bring to meal planning. Population-level surveys of amino acid intake in plant-predominant populations consistently find shortfalls in lysine, methionine, and tryptophan compared to omnivorous populations.

Digestibility — Why Grams Are Not Enough

The Protein Digestibility Corrected Amino Acid Score (PDCAAS) and its successor the Digestible Indispensable Amino Acid Score (DIAAS) are the current standard methods for assessing protein quality, accounting both for amino acid composition and digestibility. Eggs score 1.0 — the maximum. Whey protein scores close to 1.0. Most plant proteins score significantly below 1.0, particularly when digestibility is properly measured using the more rigorous ileal digestibility method that the DIAAS uses rather than the faecal digestibility method of PDCAAS.

Digestibility matters because plant proteins are frequently embedded in cell walls, phytate complexes, and fiber matrices that reduce the percentage that reaches the small intestine in absorbable form. Cooking significantly improves plant protein digestibility — the traditional practices of soaking, sprouting, and fermenting legumes and grains further improve it. But even optimally prepared plant proteins reach cells at a lower rate than animal proteins, meaning that the gram-for-gram comparison of plant and animal protein understates the advantage of animal sources when amino acid delivery to cells is the relevant metric.

IV. The Conditionally Essential Amino Acids — Where Modern Diets Fall Short

Glycine — The Most Underconsumed Structural Nutrient

Glycine's story has been told in the Structural Architects chapter and the Methylation Network chapter — it is a theme that recurs because glycine's roles are so numerous that almost every system in the book depends on it. What has not yet been fully articulated is how dramatically the modern diet has reduced glycine intake compared to traditional diets.

Traditional diets consumed the whole animal: skin (rich in collagen, therefore glycine and proline), bone broth (glycine-rich from collagen dissolution during long cooking), organ meats, and cartilaginous cuts. The modern diet in wealthy countries is dominated by skeletal muscle meat — chicken breast and other lean muscle meats — which is protein-rich but glycine-poor. The parts of the animal richest in glycine are the parts the modern diet discards.

A systematic gap has opened between glycine synthesis capacity (approximately 3g/day) and glycine requirement for optimal collagen synthesis, glutathione production, bile acid conjugation, and creatine synthesis (estimated 10–15g/day). Supplemental glycine at 3–10g/day has demonstrated clinical benefits in sleep quality, metabolic syndrome, inflammatory bowel disease, and cognitive function in clinical trials — consistent with a broad functional insufficiency whose symptomatic fingerprints are diffuse and therefore never attributed to their source.

Glutamine — The Contingency Fuel

Glutamine is the most abundant free amino acid in the human body, constituting approximately sixty percent of the free amino acid pool in muscle. Under normal conditions, the body produces enough glutamine for baseline needs. Under conditions of physiological stress — surgery, critical illness, intensive exercise, burns, or sepsis — glutamine demand from rapidly dividing cells (enterocytes, immune cells) exceeds synthesis capacity, producing a functional deficiency. This is why glutamine supplementation has been studied in surgical and critical care — the evidence demonstrates reduced infection rates, shorter hospital stays, and improved gut barrier function in patients receiving supplemental glutamine during periods of high demand.

The clinical message is that the threshold between adequate and insufficient glutamine is not fixed — it shifts dramatically under stress, illness, and intensive training. A person who is glutamine-sufficient under baseline conditions may become functionally glutamine-deficient during a significant illness or in the prolonged aftermath of surgery. This dynamic deficit is invisible to any standard blood panel and is rarely addressed in clinical practice outside of intensive care.

Cysteine and Taurine — The Sulfur Amino Acids

Cysteine is synthesized from methionine via the transsulfuration pathway (B6-dependent) and is the rate-limiting precursor for glutathione. The synthesis rate is sufficient under baseline conditions but frequently insufficient under conditions of high oxidative stress, high methionine intake without adequate B6, or inadequate dietary methionine. N-acetylcysteine (NAC) — the pharmaceutical cysteine donor — is used clinically to restore glutathione in acetaminophen overdose, in contrast dye nephropathy prevention, and in respiratory conditions. Its broader use as a glutathione support agent in individuals with high oxidative stress is supported by the same biochemistry.

Taurine — synthesized from cysteine — is the most abundant free amino acid in heart muscle, retina, brain, and skeletal muscle. It is required for bile acid conjugation (as taurocholate and taurochenodeoxycholate), for retinal protection, for cardiac rhythm regulation (modulating intracellular calcium handling), and for neurological osmoregulation. Taurine is absent from plant foods — it is found exclusively in animal products, particularly seafood and dark meat poultry. Vegans have significantly lower plasma taurine concentrations than omnivores, and the clinical consequences of this difference — in terms of cardiovascular function, retinal health, and neurological function — are incompletely understood but biochemically plausible.

Arginine and Citrulline — The Nitric Oxide Partnership

Arginine is the sole substrate for nitric oxide synthase, the enzyme that produces the nitric oxide responsible for vascular tone, endothelial function, and blood flow regulation throughout the body — connecting this chapter directly to the arterial wall integrity discussed in the Structural Architects chapter. Arginine is also the entry point to the urea cycle, the pathway that converts metabolic ammonia into urea for safe excretion — a function this book's Detoxification Network chapter depends on. Under baseline conditions, endogenous synthesis meets demand. Under cardiovascular strain, trauma, sepsis, or intensive training, requirement outstrips supply, producing a functional insufficiency that shows up as impaired vasodilation and, in critical illness, as impaired wound healing and immune function.

The clinical picture is complicated by a detail that is rarely explained to patients: dietary and supplemental arginine is heavily degraded by arginase enzymes in the intestine and liver before it ever reaches systemic circulation. Citrulline — a related compound that is not itself incorporated into protein — largely bypasses this first-pass metabolism and is converted to arginine primarily in the kidneys, often raising blood arginine levels more reliably than arginine supplementation itself. This is why citrulline, not arginine, has become the preferred clinical and research tool for restoring nitric oxide production — a case study in how the most direct-sounding intervention is not always the most effective one.

Arginine's connection to vascular health places it alongside the other quietly cardiovascular threads running through this book — copper's role in arterial wall integrity, omega-3's influence on inflammatory tone, vitamin K2's direction of calcium away from the arteries. None of these appear in a chapter titled "cardiovascular," and neither does this one. That absence is not an oversight. It is the argument.

V. Completing the Twenty

This chapter has given individual attention to fourteen amino acids and related compounds: the nine the body cannot make at all, and five — glycine, glutamine, cysteine, taurine, and arginine — whose conditional insufficiency is common enough and consequential enough to warrant it. Two more conditionally essential amino acids appear elsewhere in this book, where their clinical story is strongest: proline, which forms the structural kinks in the collagen helix, is covered in the Structural Architects chapter alongside glycine; tyrosine, the amino acid backbone of thyroid hormone, is covered in the Hormonal Regulators chapter. Their absence from this chapter's roster reflects placement, not omission.

The remaining five amino acids — alanine, aspartate, asparagine, glutamate, and serine — do not appear in this book at all. The body synthesizes all five in ample supply under ordinary conditions, and no meaningful body of evidence documents a clinical insufficiency syndrome for any of them, even under the same stressors that create functional gaps in the amino acids covered above. Twenty amino acids build every protein in the human body. Fifteen of them appear somewhere in this book, because fifteen of them have a documented capacity to run short. The other five do not, and that is itself informative: not every biological necessity is a clinical vulnerability.

VI. Amino Acids and Neurotransmitters — The Direct Connection

The connection between amino acid intake and neurotransmitter production is one of the most direct and most underappreciated nutrient-brain relationships in the book. Every major neurotransmitter is either synthesized directly from an amino acid or requires an amino acid as its immediate precursor:

Serotonin: from tryptophan (via 5-HTP, requiring iron and B6)

Dopamine, noradrenaline, adrenaline: from phenylalanine → tyrosine (requiring iron, copper, B6, vitamin C)

GABA: from glutamate (requiring B6 for glutamate decarboxylase)

Acetylcholine: requires choline (from phosphatidylcholine hydrolysis or direct dietary intake)

Histamine: from histidine (a clinically relevant connection in histamine intolerance)

Glycine and taurine: directly function as inhibitory neurotransmitters in the spinal cord and brainstem

A psychiatric patient whose amino acid intake, digestibility, and competition at the blood-brain barrier transporters have never been assessed is a patient whose neurotransmitter production capacity is entirely opaque to the clinicians managing their mood. The medications prescribed adjust the availability of neurotransmitters that have already been produced. The nutritional foundation of that production is invisible.

VII. The Web of Dependencies

Amino acids underpin all other clusters: Collagen requires glycine, proline, lysine (Cluster 5). Glutathione requires glycine, cysteine, glutamate (Cluster 4). Neurotransmitters require tryptophan, tyrosine, histidine (Cluster 7). Methylation requires methionine (Cluster 9). Detoxification requires glycine, taurine, glutamine, cysteine (Cluster 10). The amino acid cluster is the foundational material supplier for the entire orchestra.

Gut determines what is available: The gut (Cluster 2) determines amino acid digestibility and absorption. A damaged gut lining may absorb dietary protein poorly — producing adequate protein intake by weight but inadequate amino acid delivery to cells. The gut's own highest-priority amino acid demand is for glutamine and threonine, meaning that gut damage and amino acid insufficiency create a self-reinforcing cycle.

Iron and B6 enable the conversions: Tryptophan cannot become serotonin without iron and B6. Phenylalanine cannot become dopamine without iron, copper, B6, and vitamin C. The amino acid provides the raw material; the micronutrients from other clusters perform the conversion. Without both, the synthesis chain stalls.

> *The person prescribed an antidepressant because serotonin is insufficient is being given a drug that prevents the reuptake of serotonin that has already been produced — from tryptophan that was available, absorbed through a gut that was functioning, converted by enzymes that had adequate iron and B6 cofactors. Prescribe the drug without asking whether any of these conditions are met, and you are adjusting the availability of a neurotransmitter whose production*

> *you have never looked at. The upstream goes uninvestigated. The downstream gets medicated. The pattern holds.*

VIII. Questions Worth Asking

For a person with muscle wasting, persistent fatigue, poor wound healing, recurrent infections, mood instability, or unexplained digestive symptoms — the amino acid foundation represents a genuinely assessable upstream territory.

Plasma amino acid profiles measure the free amino acid pool and can identify specific deficiencies that dietary assessment would miss. Urinary amino acid excretion can reveal renal tubular reabsorption problems. Serum albumin and prealbumin provide gross markers of protein status (though they are affected by inflammation). Hair mineral analysis, while limited in scope, can suggest protein adequacy from hair growth patterns. Dietary recall focused specifically on amino acid sources — not just protein grams — can identify compositional gaps in plant-predominant diets.

The information in this chapter is educational and does not constitute clinical advice. Dietary changes, particularly in protein composition, should be considered in the context of the individual's full health status, including kidney function, which may limit protein intake in some individuals. The author does not offer clinical recommendations for any individual.

For the Clinically Curious

mTOR and Leucine — The Anabolic Signaling Mechanism

Leucine activates mammalian target of rapamycin complex 1 (mTORC1) through a mechanism involving the Ragulator-Rag GTPase complex on the lysosomal surface and the upstream leucine sensor Sestrin2. mTORC1 activation phosphorylates S6 kinase 1 (S6K1) and eukaryotic initiation factor 4E-binding protein 1 (4EBP1), driving ribosomal biogenesis and translation initiation for muscle protein synthesis. The threshold leucine concentration required for mTORC1 activation differs between young and older adults — older adults require higher per-meal leucine concentrations (typically above 2–3g per meal) to achieve the same anabolic response, explaining the blunted muscle protein synthesis rate in aging populations even with adequate total protein intake. This leucine threshold effect means that distribution of protein across meals matters: three meals each containing adequate leucine produce more cumulative muscle protein synthesis than six smaller meals or one large meal with the same total protein.

Plasma Amino Acid Analysis — Clinical Interpretation

Plasma amino acid analysis measures the free amino acid pool, which reflects the balance between dietary intake, endogenous synthesis, tissue protein turnover, and utilization for biosynthesis. Reference ranges are established for fasting plasma; post-prandial samples reflect recent intake. Key clinical patterns: low tryptophan with high kynurenine/tryptophan ratio indicates IDO-mediated diversion toward the kynurenine pathway, seen in systemic inflammation and associated with depression; low glycine with normal total protein suggests inadequate collagen-type dietary protein sources; elevated homocysteine (measured separately) alongside low methionine suggests impaired methionine recycling through the methylation cycle; low glutamine in the context of illness, surgery, or intensive training indicates depletion of the contingency fuel reserve.

Taurine and Cardiac Function — The Evidence Base

Taurine is the most abundant amino acid in cardiac muscle (10–40 mM intracellular concentration) where it regulates calcium handling, protects against oxidative stress, and modulates cardiac contractility through its interaction with the ryanodine receptor and SERCA calcium pumps. Taurine deficiency produces dilated cardiomyopathy in cats (who cannot synthesize taurine at all) and was identified in 2018 as the cause of diet-associated dilated cardiomyopathy in dogs fed grain-free diets — a canine model with direct implications for taurine's role in human cardiac health. Population studies show that higher dietary taurine intake (from seafood consumption) is associated with lower cardiovascular mortality. A 2020 systematic review found that taurine supplementation significantly reduced blood pressure in hypertensive subjects and improved cardiac function markers. The consistent taurine depletion in vegans represents a cardiovascular risk factor that is essentially never discussed in the clinical management of plant-based dieters.

Cluster 12

The Fat-Soluble Foundations

How Vitamins A, D, E, K, and Cholesterol Form the Body's Regulatory and Structural Fat-Soluble System — and Why Their Interdependency Is More Important Than Any of Them Alone

> *"The fat-soluble vitamins are not a shopping list. They are a system — four conductors who share a stage and cannot perform without one another present."*

I. The Vitamins That Disappeared With Fat

There is a historical irony at the center of the fat-soluble vitamin story. The public health advice that dominated the second half of the twentieth century — reduce dietary fat, choose low-fat products, avoid egg yolks, limit red meat — removed from the diet precisely the foods richest in the fat-soluble vitamins that the nutrients' very name describes. Vitamins A, D, E, and K are fat-soluble. They are found in fat-containing foods. When fat was removed from food, or when fat-containing foods were replaced by carbohydrate-heavy alternatives, the fat-soluble vitamins went with them.

The fat-phobic dietary era ran from approximately 1970 to 2010. Four decades during which populations were systematically steered away from butter (vitamin A, D, K2), egg yolks (A, D, E, K), liver (A, D, K), whole milk (A, D, K2), fatty fish (D, E, omega-3), and cheese (A, D, K2). The nutritional consequences of that steering are still being calculated. The fat-soluble vitamin insufficiency epidemic — the measurable decline in population levels of vitamins A, D, E, and K2 documented across multiple countries in the low-fat era — represents one of the most consequential and least acknowledged public health failures of the modern age.

II. Meet the Cast

Six principal members form the fat-soluble regulatory system — four vitamins, the phospholipid membrane backbone that enables their function, and one molecule that medicine mistakenly classified as a cardiovascular risk factor:

- **Vitamin A (retinol and retinoids)** — The master regulator of cell differentiation — determining whether stem cells become epithelial cells, immune cells, reproductive cells, or neurons. Acts through retinoic acid receptors (RAR) and retinoid X receptors (RXR) that partner with virtually every other nuclear receptor in the body.
- **Vitamin D (cholecalciferol and calcitriol)** — The solar hormone — structurally a steroid hormone, not a vitamin.

Acts through vitamin D receptors (VDR) expressed in virtually every tissue, regulating over 2,000 genes involved in immunity, calcium metabolism, cell growth, and inflammation.

- **Vitamin E (tocopherols and tocotrienols)** — The membrane-resident antioxidant — fat-soluble, embedded in cell membranes, protecting polyunsaturated fatty acids from lipid peroxidation. Eight distinct forms with different potencies and tissue distributions.
- **Vitamin K1 and K2** — K1 (phylloquinone) governs blood clotting through carboxylation of clotting factors. K2 (menaquinones, particularly MK-4 and MK-7) governs calcium routing through carboxylation of matrix Gla protein and osteocalcin — directing calcium into bone and away from arteries.
- **Phosphorus (as phospholipids)** — The Membrane Backbone. The structural scaffold on which every fat-soluble vitamin acts. Phosphatidylcholine, phosphatidylserine, and sphingomyelin provide the lipid bilayer that every fat-soluble molecule traverses and every membrane receptor inhabits.
- **Cholesterol** — The structural precursor of all steroid hormones (cortisol, testosterone, estrogen, aldosterone), vitamin D, and bile acids. The molecule that medicine spent five decades demonising is the molecule from which the body's entire steroid hormone and fat-soluble vitamin system is constructed.

III. Vitamin A — The Master Differentiator

Retinol vs. Beta-Carotene: The Conversion Problem

Vitamin A exists in two dietary forms: preformed retinol (in animal products — liver, eggs, dairy, fatty fish) and provitamin A carotenoids (primarily beta-carotene, in plant foods). They are not equivalent. Retinol is immediately bioavailable. Beta-carotene must be converted to retinol by the enzyme beta-carotene 15,15'-monooxygenase 1 (BCMO1), and this conversion is variable, incomplete, and affected by multiple factors including genetic variants in the BCMO1 gene.

Approximately forty-five percent of people carry common BCMO1 variants that reduce beta-carotene conversion efficiency by fifty to seventy percent. These individuals cannot reliably meet their vitamin A needs from plant sources regardless of how many carrots they eat. For them, preformed retinol from animal sources is functionally essential — the plant-based vitamin A story simply does not work. This genetic reality has been documented but is essentially absent from public health vitamin A guidance, which treats beta-carotene and retinol as equivalent — which, for a significant fraction of the population, they are not.

What Retinol Actually Does

Vitamin A — as retinoic acid — operates through the most extensive nuclear receptor signaling system in human biology. Retinoic acid receptors (RAR-alpha, -beta, -gamma) and retinoid X receptors (RXR-alpha, -beta, -gamma) form homo- and heterodimers that bind retinoic acid response elements (RAREs) in the regulatory regions of hundreds of genes. RXR partners not only with RAR but with the vitamin D receptor (VDR), the thyroid hormone receptor (THR), the peroxisome proliferator-activated receptors (PPARs), and the liver X receptors (LXR) — meaning that adequate vitamin A is required for full signaling through these other nuclear receptors as well.

The practical consequences of vitamin A deficiency are among the most dramatic of any micronutrient: night blindness (rhodopsin in rod photoreceptors requires 11-cis-retinal), xerophthalmia (the drying and thickening of the conjunctiva and cornea), impaired immune defense at mucosal surfaces, impaired embryonic development (retinoic acid is required for limb and organ morphogenesis), and impaired cell differentiation throughout the body. Subclinical vitamin A insufficiency — below the threshold of clinical deficiency — produces impaired mucosal immunity, increased infection susceptibility, and dysregulated cell differentiation that is invisible to standard clinical assessment.

Toxicity — Separating Fact from Fear

Vitamin A has a legitimate toxicity concern — excessive preformed retinol produces hypervitaminosis A, with symptoms including headache, nausea, bone pain, and, at very high doses, liver damage. Teratogenicity at doses above 10,000 IU/day in pregnancy is documented (Rothman et al., New England Journal of Medicine, 1995). These concerns are real and justify caution with high-dose supplementation in pregnancy.

What is not justified is the extrapolation of toxicity risk from pharmacological doses to dietary and moderate supplemental doses. The doses that produce toxicity in most reported cases are ten to one hundred times the dose required for nutritional sufficiency. The fear of vitamin A toxicity has produced unnecessary avoidance of liver consumption (the world's most nutrient-dense food) and unnecessary limitation of vitamin A supplementation in populations where deficiency is prevalent. The dose makes the poison — and the doses required for adequacy are far removed from the doses associated with toxicity.

IV. Vitamin D — The Solar Hormone

Structure and Function

Vitamin D is structurally a secosteroid — a steroid with a broken B ring — and behaves pharmacologically as a hormone rather than a cofactor. It is produced in skin from 7-dehydrocholesterol under UVB radiation (wavelengths 290–315 nm), hydroxylated in the liver to 25(OH)D (the storage form measured in blood), and then hydroxylated again in the kidney and in peripheral tissues to the active 1,25(OH)2D (calcitriol). This final step is regulated by PTH and serum calcium, creating a hormonal axis — not a simple dietary supplement pathway.

The vitamin D receptor is expressed in over thirty tissue types, and genome-wide analysis has identified over 2,000 genes as potential vitamin D targets. The vitamin D-regulated genes include those involved in immune regulation (described in Cluster 8), calcium metabolism, cell proliferation and differentiation, insulin secretion, and neurological function. Vitamin D is not a calcium vitamin with some additional properties. It is a systemic regulatory hormone with calcium metabolism as one of its many functions.

The Epidemic That Medicine Created

Global recommendations to avoid sun exposure — motivated by skin cancer prevention — and the architectural and lifestyle changes of modern life (indoor work, indoor living, glass-filtered sunlight that blocks UVB) have produced a population-scale vitamin D deficiency that is among the most preventable micronutrient epidemics in history. Surveys across Europe, North America, Asia, and the Middle East consistently find that fifty to eighty percent of population samples have 25(OH)D concentrations below 30 ng/mL — the threshold commonly used to define insufficiency. In some populations, particularly those with darker skin at higher latitudes, rates of frank deficiency (below 20 ng/mL) exceed fifty percent.

The consequences are not limited to calcium metabolism and bone health. The epidemiological associations between vitamin D deficiency and autoimmune disease (multiple sclerosis, rheumatoid arthritis, type 1 diabetes, inflammatory bowel disease), cardiovascular disease, respiratory infections, mood disorders, and cancer risk have been documented across hundreds of studies. The mechanistic basis — vitamin D's role in immune regulation, inflammation modulation, cell differentiation, and neurotransmitter synthesis — is established. The clinical translation — routine assessment and correction of vitamin D status as a component of management for these conditions — has been glacially slow.

The Cofactor Web

Vitamin D supplementation in isolation frequently underperforms its theoretical benefit, and the reason is the cofactor web that vitamin D requires to function fully. Magnesium is required for the enzymatic hydroxylation steps that activate vitamin D — both the 25-hydroxylation in the liver and the 1-alpha-hydroxylation in the kidney and peripheral tissues use magnesium-dependent hydroxylases. A person with magnesium deficiency supplementing vitamin D may raise their 25(OH)D level while still having impaired conversion to the active 1,25(OH)2D. Vitamin A is required for full VDR signaling — the VDR-RXR heterodimer requires both vitamin D and retinoic acid for optimal DNA binding. Vitamin K2 is required to prevent hypercalcemia and soft tissue calcification that can result from aggressive vitamin D supplementation without adequate calcium routing. The four fat-soluble vitamins are not independent — they are a system that must be supported together.

V. Vitamin K1 and K2 — Two Different Jobs

K1 — The Clotting Vitamin

Vitamin K1 (phylloquinone) is found in leafy green vegetables and activates the clotting factors II, VII, IX, X, and the anticoagulant proteins C and S through gamma-carboxylation of glutamate residues. This is the vitamin K that anticoagulant medications (warfarin, acenocoumarol) target — they block vitamin K recycling, reducing clotting factor carboxylation and reducing clotting capacity. K1 is generally adequately supplied in green-vegetable-containing diets and is rarely clinically deficient in adults outside of fat malabsorption syndromes.

K2 — The Calcium Director

Vitamin K2 — the menaquinones, particularly MK-4 (found in animal foods) and MK-7 (found in fermented foods, particularly natto) — activates matrix Gla protein (MGP) and osteocalcin through the same gamma-carboxylation mechanism. As described in Cluster 5, activated MGP prevents arterial calcification; activated osteocalcin enables calcium binding to bone matrix. K2 and K1 are handled differently by the body: K1 is rapidly cleared from the circulation; K2 (particularly the long-chain MK-7 form) has a much longer half-life and reaches peripheral tissues including bone and arterial walls where its calcium-directing function is performed.

K2 is the fat-soluble vitamin most dramatically reduced by the low-fat dietary era. Its primary dietary sources — fermented dairy, natto, goose liver pâté, hard cheeses, egg yolks, butter from grass-fed animals — are precisely the foods that were discouraged by two generations of low-fat dietary advice. The Rotterdam Study's finding of fifty-seven percent lower cardiovascular mortality in the highest K2 intake quartile versus the lowest represents one of the most dramatic and least discussed diet-disease associations in the cardiovascular literature.

VI. Cholesterol — The Vilified Building Block

Cholesterol is the precursor from which the body synthesizes all steroid hormones (cortisol, testosterone, oestradiol, progesterone, DHEA, aldosterone), vitamin D (from 7-dehydrocholesterol), and bile acids (required for fat digestion and fat-soluble vitamin absorption). It is also a structural component of every cell membrane in the body, where it modulates membrane fluidity and provides the scaffold on which membrane-bound proteins are organized.

The dietary cholesterol-cardiovascular disease hypothesis — that eating cholesterol raises blood cholesterol and causes heart disease — has been significantly revised over the past two decades. Dietary cholesterol has been removed from the list of 'nutrients of concern' in the 2015 US Dietary Guidelines, reflecting the evidence that dietary cholesterol has minimal effect on cardiovascular risk in most people and that endogenous synthesis (which produces approximately eighty percent of total body cholesterol) is the primary determinant of blood cholesterol levels.

The practical consequence of the cholesterol-phobic dietary era for fat-soluble nutrition was significant: eggs — one of nature's most nutrient-complete foods, rich in vitamins A, D, E, K2, choline, and every essential amino acid — were restricted. Liver — the single richest dietary source of vitamins A, D, B12, folate, iron, and copper — was discouraged. Whole dairy — a source of vitamins A, D, K2, and calcium — was replaced by fat-free versions stripped of fat-soluble vitamins. The nutritional collateral damage of cholesterol avoidance extended well beyond cholesterol itself.

VII. Phosphorus — The Membrane's Invisible Foundation

Every fat-soluble vitamin in this chapter — A, D, E, and K — is absorbed into, transported through, and inserted into cell membranes that are built on a phospholipid scaffold. Phosphatidylcholine, phosphatidylethanolamine, phosphatidylserine, sphingomyelin — the phospholipids of the bilayer — are all phosphate-containing lipids. The phosphate group provides the polar head that faces the aqueous environment on both sides of the membrane; the fatty acid tails face inward, creating the bilayer that separates the cell interior from the exterior world. Remove the phosphate and the membrane loses its amphipathic character entirely. Every fat-soluble vitamin described in this chapter requires the phospholipid membrane for its absorption from the gut, its transport through the lymphatic and circulatory system, and its functional integration at nuclear receptors and cell membrane signaling complexes throughout the body.

Phosphatidylserine — the phospholipid concentrated on the inner leaflet of neuronal plasma membranes — has documented roles in cognitive function, memory consolidation, and stress response modulation through its influence on cortisol regulation. Phosphatidylcholine is the structural carrier for DHA in neuronal membranes: DHA reaches the brain incorporated into phosphatidylcholine-DHA, making phosphorus and choline jointly necessary for DHA's neurological structural function. The fat-soluble vitamin system of this cluster and the essential fatty acid system of Cluster 13 are both phospholipid-dependent. Neither can be fully understood without recognizing phosphorus as the invisible structural backbone on which both operate.

Its essential partners: *Phospholipid synthesis requires choline (for phosphatidylcholine), serine (for phosphatidylserine), and the omega-3 fatty acids of Cluster 13 — particularly DHA, which is incorporated as phosphatidylcholine-DHA into neuronal membranes. The methylation network (Cluster 9) provides methyl groups for phosphatidylcholine synthesis via the PEMT pathway. The quality of the membrane is therefore a function of phosphorus adequacy, choline supply, omega-3 fatty acid status, and methylation network function simultaneously — making phospholipid membranes the single most cross-referenced molecular structure in this book.*

VIII. The Fat-Soluble System's Interdependencies

No other cluster in this book has more documented nutrient-nutrient interactions than the fat-soluble group:

Vitamin A and D share RXR: The retinoid X receptor (RXR) is required by both vitamin A (as a RAR-RXR heterodimer) and vitamin D (as a VDR-RXR heterodimer). When both vitamins are adequate, each activates its respective receptor system fully. When vitamin A is insufficient, RXR availability for VDR signaling may be reduced — impairing vitamin D's function at the receptor level even when

25(OH)D is adequate. Conversely, excessive vitamin A may compete with vitamin D for RXR and impair vitamin D receptor signaling.

Vitamin D drives calcium; vitamin K2 routes it: Vitamin D increases intestinal calcium absorption and raises circulating calcium. Vitamin K2 activates the proteins (MGP and osteocalcin) that direct that calcium into bone and prevent it from depositing in arterial walls. Without K2, aggressive vitamin D supplementation increases the risk of arterial calcification. The D-K2 pair must be understood together.

Vitamin E requires vitamin C: After neutralizing a lipid peroxyl radical in the membrane, vitamin E (tocopherol) becomes a tocopheroxyl radical that is regenerated by vitamin C. In vitamin C-depleted states, vitamin E cannot be recycled and is consumed irreversibly, accelerating its depletion. The fat-soluble and water-soluble antioxidant networks are coupled.

All four require fat for absorption: Vitamins A, D, E, and K are only absorbed in the presence of dietary fat. Low-fat meals produce significantly lower absorption of all four. The dietary fat that the low-fat era removed was not only a source of these vitamins but the vehicle for their absorption.

> *The fat-soluble vitamins were removed from the diet by advice designed to prevent heart disease. The advice was wrong about fat's role in heart disease, and the*

> *nutritional collateral damage — the vitamins A, D, E, and K2 that went with the fat — may have contributed to the very conditions the advice was meant to prevent. Arterial calcification (which adequate K2 prevents), impaired immunity (which adequate D prevents), increased cancer risk (which adequate A modulates), and accelerated oxidative damage to arterial membranes (which adequate E prevents) are all conditions the fat-phobic era potentially worsened while trying to improve cardiovascular outcomes.*

IX. Questions Worth Asking

A comprehensive fat-soluble assessment includes: 25(OH)D with PTH and magnesium (for functional vitamin D status); serum retinol with RBP4 (retinol-binding protein, which transports retinol — low RBP4 indicates vitamin A deficiency regardless of serum retinol); undercarboxylated osteocalcin and undercarboxylated MGP for K2 functional status; plasma alpha-tocopherol corrected for total lipids for vitamin E status.

The information in this chapter is educational and does not constitute clinical advice. Vitamin A supplementation in pregnancy requires medical supervision given documented teratogenicity at high doses. Vitamin D supplementation above standard doses should be monitored with blood testing for 25(OH)D and calcium. Any changes to anticoagulant medication in the context of vitamin K supplementation must be managed by a qualified clinician. The author does not offer clinical recommendations.

For the Clinically Curious

RXR as the Nuclear Receptor Hub — Clinical Implications

Retinoid X receptor (RXR) forms obligate heterodimers with over a dozen nuclear receptors: RAR (retinoic acid receptor), VDR (vitamin D receptor), THR (thyroid hormone receptor), PPAR-alpha and gamma (metabolic regulators), LXR (liver X receptor, regulating cholesterol metabolism), FXR (farnesoid X receptor, regulating bile acid metabolism), and others. This RXR dependence means that adequate vitamin A availability modulates the signaling of all these systems simultaneously. Clinical implications: vitamin A deficiency impairs thyroid hormone receptor signaling (contributing to hypothyroid symptoms), impairs PPAR-gamma signaling (contributing to insulin resistance), and impairs LXR signaling (affecting cholesterol metabolism) — independent of the specific effects of thyroid hormone, insulin, or cholesterol levels themselves. This cross-receptor role of RXR makes vitamin A sufficiency a prerequisite for the full function of multiple hormonal systems that standard medicine treats as independent.

Menaquinone-7 (MK-7) Pharmacokinetics and Clinical Evidence

MK-7, the long-chain menaquinone form of K2 found predominantly in natto and produced in smaller quantities by other fermented foods, has a plasma half-life of approximately 72 hours compared to approximately 1-2 hours for vitamin K1. This extended half-life allows once-daily dosing and enables MK-7 to reach peripheral tissues including bone and arterial walls, where MK-4 (the short-chain form from animal foods) also accumulates through active tissue uptake. The clinical K2 evidence base is primarily from European cohort studies and Dutch investigations, including: the Rotterdam Study (Geleijnse et al., 2004) showing 57% lower cardiovascular mortality and 26% lower coronary calcification in highest menaquinone tertile; the Prospect-EPIC cohort showing K2 association with lower aortic calcification and cardiovascular events; and multiple bone mineral density trials showing MK-7 preservation of bone mineral density in postmenopausal women. Standard recommended intake for K2 remains undefined in most countries; observed intake in high-natto-consuming Japanese populations (>250 mcg/day) differs dramatically from typical Western intake (<10 mcg/day).

Tocotrienols — The Understudied Vitamin E Forms

Alpha-tocopherol has dominated vitamin E research and supplementation, while the tocotrienol forms (alpha-, beta-, gamma-, delta-tocotrienols) have received less clinical attention despite possessing distinct — and in some respects superior — biological properties. Tocotrienols move more freely within membranes due to their unsaturated isoprenoid side chain (tocopherols have a saturated phytyl chain), providing potentially superior distribution in neuronal membranes. Delta-tocotrienol has demonstrated anti-cancer properties in multiple cell and animal models, particularly for pancreatic cancer. Gamma-tocotrienol inhibits HMG-CoA reductase (the same enzyme targeted by statins), providing a natural cholesterol-lowering mechanism. Palm oil and rice bran oil are the richest dietary sources. The clinical evidence for tocotrienols remains less developed than for tocopherols, but their unique biological properties distinguish them from alpha-tocopherol in ways that warrant attention in the vitamin E therapeutic literature.

Cluster 13

The Essential Fatty Acids

How the Balance Between Omega-3 and Omega-6 Fats Governs Inflammation, Brain Architecture, Cardiovascular Health, and Cell Signaling — and Why the Most Important Dietary Change of the Last Century Was an Accident Nobody Noticed

"We changed the fat in our food, and we changed the fat in our cells. Nobody planned it. Nobody announced it. Nobody measured what it meant. We are still paying."

I. The Accidental Experiment

Between approximately 1960 and 2000, the Western food supply underwent a transformation in its fat composition that was without precedent in human evolutionary history. Traditional animal fats — butter, tallow, and the fat in pasture-raised meat — were displaced by industrially produced vegetable oils: soybean oil, corn oil, cottonseed oil, sunflower oil, and eventually canola oil. These oils are rich in linoleic acid — an omega-6 polyunsaturated fat — and were promoted as heart-healthy alternatives to saturated animal fats. They were cheap to produce, shelf-stable when partially hydrogenated, and backed by dietary guidelines that identified saturated fat as the dietary villain in cardiovascular disease.

The omega-6 content of the modern Western diet rose from approximately two percent of caloric intake in 1900 to approximately eight percent by 2010 — a four-fold increase. The ratio of omega-6 to omega-3 fatty acids in the diet shifted from an estimated ancestral ratio of approximately 4:1 to the current 15:1 to 20:1. This shift was not a nutrient deficiency in the traditional sense — no individual was acutely deficient in omega-3 fatty acids. It was a systemic compositional change in the fat profile of the human body, producing cells, membranes, and tissues with a fundamentally different fatty acid architecture than any that had existed in prior human history.

No clinical trial was run. No safety assessment was conducted. No population monitoring measured the consequences over time. The experiment was conducted on an entire civilisation, without controls, without follow-up, and without the recognition that changing the fat in food changes the fat in cells — including the cells of the brain, the heart, the immune system, and the arterial wall.

II. Meet the Cast

The essential fatty acid orchestra has four principal families — omega-3, omega-6, omega-9, and the ratio between the first two that governs their biological effects. Seven key members are listed here, followed by a note on the ratio that ties them together:

- **ALA (alpha-linolenic acid) — omega-3** — The short-chain omega-3 essential fatty acid found in flaxseed, walnuts, chia, and hemp. The body can convert ALA to EPA and DHA but with very low efficiency (typically one to five percent), making ALA a poor substitute for preformed EPA and DHA from marine sources.
- **EPA (eicosapentaenoic acid) — omega-3** — The twenty-carbon omega-3 found in fatty fish, shellfish, and algae. The primary precursor to anti-inflammatory eicosanoids and E-series resolvins. Modulates neuroinflammation, prostaglandin balance, and platelet aggregation.
- **DHA (docosahexaenoic acid) — omega-3** — The twenty-two-carbon omega-3, structurally dominant in neuronal membranes (approximately sixty percent of brain structural fat), photoreceptor membranes, and cardiac muscle. The primary determinant of neuronal membrane fluidity and receptor dynamics.
- **LA (linoleic acid) — omega-6** — The short-chain omega-6 essential fatty acid found in virtually all vegetable oils and most seeds. Required in modest quantities. In modern diets, present in quantities that dwarf any ancestral exposure.
- **GLA (gamma-linolenic acid) — omega-6** — The elongated omega-6 produced from LA by delta-6-desaturase. Found in evening primrose oil, borage oil, and blackcurrant seed oil. Has anti-inflammatory properties distinct from other

omega-6 fatty acids, producing the anti-inflammatory prostaglandin E1 series via DGLA.

- **AA (arachidonic acid) — omega-6** — The twenty-carbon omega-6 derived from DGLA. The primary precursor to pro-inflammatory eicosanoids (prostaglandin E2, leukotriene B4, thromboxane A2) that initiate and amplify inflammation. Essential for immune function and for neural development — but damaging when imbalanced against omega-3.
- **Oleic acid — omega-9** — The primary monounsaturated fat in olive oil, avocado, and almonds. Not essential (the body can synthesize it) but anti-inflammatory, resistant to oxidation, and the fat most associated with Mediterranean diet benefits. Competes favorably with omega-6 in membranes.
- **The omega-3:omega-6 ratio** — Not a single nutrient but the most clinically important number in the essential fatty acid story — the balance between the two families that determines the body's basal inflammatory tone.

III. How Fatty Acids Govern Inflammation

The Eicosanoid Cascade — Two Directions

Omega-6 and omega-3 fatty acids compete for the same enzymes — cyclooxygenase (COX) and lipoxygenase (LOX) — that convert them to eicosanoids: prostaglandins, thromboxanes, and leukotrienes that mediate inflammation, clotting, immune activation, and vascular tone. The substrates fed into these enzymes determine whether the output is inflammatory or resolving.

Arachidonic acid (omega-6) fed to COX produces prostaglandin E2 (PGE2) — a potent pro-inflammatory signaling molecule that dilates blood vessels, sensitizes pain receptors, promotes immune cell recruitment, and raises body temperature. PGE2 is not inherently bad — it is a required component of the acute inflammatory response that enables healing. The problem is chronic PGE2 production driven by a membrane AA pool that vastly exceeds what normal immune function requires.

EPA (omega-3) fed to the same COX enzyme produces prostaglandin E3 (PGE3) — a substantially less potent inflammatory mediator that competes with PGE2 for receptor binding, producing a net reduction in inflammatory signaling. EPA also generates the E-series resolvins — bioactive molecules that actively resolve inflammation by promoting clearance of inflammatory debris and suppressing neutrophil recruitment. DHA generates D-series resolvins and protectins with analogous resolution functions.

The dietary ratio of omega-6 to omega-3 therefore directly determines the prostaglandin balance in every tissue of the body. A diet with a 15:1 ratio produces cells whose membrane AA to EPA ratio results in dramatically more PGE2 and less PGE3 than cells from a diet with a 4:1 ratio — creating a systemic inflammatory baseline that is elevated by dietary composition rather than by any pathological trigger. This is not acute inflammation. It is a permanently elevated inflammatory tone, maintained by the fat in the cells, driving the low-grade chronic inflammation that underpins cardiovascular disease, metabolic syndrome, neurodegeneration, autoimmune conditions, and cancer progression.

IV. DHA and the Brain

The Architectural Fatty Acid

DHA constitutes approximately sixty percent of the brain's structural fat, concentrated primarily in the synaptic membranes where neurotransmitter receptors reside and where all neuronal signaling transactions occur. DHA is not a cofactor or a signaling molecule in the traditional sense — it is a structural component of the physical substrate on which neuronal communication depends.

Membrane DHA content determines membrane fluidity — the physical property that governs how quickly membrane proteins can move, change conformation, and interact with their partners. DHA-rich membranes are more fluid than DHA-depleted membranes. Greater fluidity means faster receptor conformational changes, more efficient neurotransmitter receptor clustering, and more rapid ion channel dynamics. The practical consequence: neuronal signaling in DHA-rich brains is physically faster and more efficient than in DHA-depleted brains.

DHA accumulates in the brain primarily during the last trimester of pregnancy and the first two years of life — the period of most rapid neural proliferation and synaptic development. Maternal DHA status during pregnancy directly determines fetal and infant brain DHA composition. Population studies have consistently found that higher maternal DHA status during pregnancy is associated with higher infant cognitive scores, better visual acuity, and superior language development. The brain's nutritional geography is partly set in utero by the fat composition of the mother's diet.

DHA in Neurodegeneration

In adults, DHA depletion in neuronal membranes is associated with accelerated cognitive decline and increased Alzheimer's disease risk. The mechanism involves multiple pathways: DHA-depleted membranes are less fluid, impairing receptor function and synaptic transmission; DHA depletion promotes amyloid precursor protein processing toward the amyloidogenic pathway; and DHA modulates neuroinflammation through its resolvin D-series metabolites, which reduce microglial inflammatory activation. Observational studies consistently find lower DHA concentrations in the brains of Alzheimer's patients compared to age-matched controls. Intervention trials with DHA supplementation have shown mixed results — more positive in populations with lower baseline DHA status and in those without established dementia — suggesting a preventive rather than therapeutic role.

V. The Seed Oil Problem

Oxidative Instability

Polyunsaturated fatty acids — the omega-6 rich linoleic acid dominant in vegetable oils — are highly susceptible to oxidative damage. Each additional double bond in the carbon chain increases reactivity with oxygen. Linoleic acid (two double bonds) is more oxidation-prone than oleic acid (one double bond) in olive oil. Arachidonic acid (four double bonds) is more reactive still. DHA (six double bonds) is the most oxidation-susceptible of all common fatty acids.

When seed oils rich in polyunsaturated fatty acids are heated — for cooking, for industrial food processing, for frying — they undergo oxidative degradation that produces aldehydes, trans fats, and cyclic fatty acid monomers that are toxic to cells at concentrations achievable through cooking use. Oxidized linoleic acid metabolites (OXLAMs) — including 4-hydroxynonenal (4-HNE) and malondialdehyde (MDA) — are genotoxic, protein-crosslinking, and mitochondria-damaging compounds detected in fried food and in the tissues of people consuming high-seed-oil diets.

Traditional cooking fats — butter, ghee, tallow, coconut oil — are predominantly saturated or monounsaturated and are therefore substantially more stable to heat than polyunsaturated seed oils. The replacement of these traditional fats with polyunsaturated vegetable oils for cooking introduced a systematic source of dietary oxidized fat products that traditional diets did not contain. The health consequences of chronic low-level exposure to dietary

OXLAMs are still being characterized, but the biochemical mechanism of harm is clearly established.

The Trans Fat Interlude

Partial hydrogenation of vegetable oils — the industrial process that converts liquid vegetable oil to solid or semi-solid margarine and shortening — produces artificial trans fatty acids: molecules with a trans rather than cis configuration at the double bond. Trans fats from partial hydrogenation are absent from nature (small amounts of natural trans fats from ruminant digestion exist in dairy, but these are structurally distinct and have different biological effects). Artificial trans fats raise LDL cholesterol, lower HDL cholesterol, increase inflammation, and are associated with cardiovascular disease risk more strongly than any other dietary fat. They were introduced into the food supply in the 1950s and 1960s as the 'healthy' alternative to saturated animal fats, and were not removed from the US food supply until 2015 — approximately sixty years of population-scale exposure to a fat the body cannot metabolize appropriately.

VI. Correcting the Ratio

The Marine Sources

EPA and DHA are found preformed in fatty fish — salmon, mackerel, sardines, herring, anchovies — and in shellfish and algae. The recommendation to consume fatty fish two to three times per week is one of the few dietary recommendations in conventional medicine with a mechanistically clear nutritional rationale: it directly raises cell membrane EPA and DHA, shifts the prostaglandin balance toward resolution, improves neuronal membrane fluidity, and reduces systemic inflammatory markers.

Fish oil supplementation delivers EPA and DHA directly without the ocean-to-table supply chain and mercury exposure concerns that limit fatty fish consumption for some populations. The evidence for fish oil supplementation in cardiovascular disease prevention was mixed in earlier trials (which used lower doses) and has improved with higher-dose trials: the REDUCE-IT trial demonstrated that high-dose EPA (4g/day as icosapentaenoic acid ethyl ester) significantly reduced cardiovascular events in statin-treated high-risk patients. The STRENGTH trial with a combination EPA/DHA product showed no benefit, suggesting that the form of omega-3 supplementation matters — a nuance absent from most clinical guidance.

The Plant-Based Alternative

ALA from flaxseed, chia, walnuts, and hemp converts to EPA at approximately five to ten percent efficiency and to DHA at approximately zero to four percent. For vegans and vegetarians, algal oil — derived from the marine algae that fish themselves eat to accumulate EPA and DHA — provides preformed EPA and DHA without the fish. Algal oil is the direct source and is in some respects more pure and more sustainably produced than fish oil. For any individual relying on plant sources for omega-3, algal oil is the essential supplement.

VII. The Web of Dependencies

Omega-3 requires vitamin E: EPA and DHA are highly polyunsaturated and vulnerable to lipid peroxidation in membranes. Vitamin E is the membrane-resident antioxidant that protects them from oxidative damage. Supplementing omega-3 without adequate vitamin E may result in the omega-3 being oxidized before it can fulfill its structural function.

Omega-3 requires zinc for resolution: The enzymes that convert EPA and DHA to resolvins and protectins include zinc-dependent metalloenzymes. The anti-inflammatory resolution function of EPA and DHA depends on adequate zinc.

DHA requires choline: Phosphatidylcholine-DHA — the primary form of DHA in neuronal membranes — requires choline as its head group. Choline deficiency limits the incorporation of DHA into the phospholipid structure that constitutes the neuronal membrane.

The ratio is more important than the absolute: Increasing omega-3 intake without reducing omega-6 intake produces partial improvement in the ratio. The most effective strategy — consistent with the evidence from Mediterranean, Japanese, and traditional diet comparisons — is both increasing omega-3 and reducing excessive omega-6 from seed oils simultaneously.

> *We did not intend to change the fat in our brains, our hearts, and our immune systems. We changed the fat in our food, and it changed us. The omega-3 to omega-6 ratio in Western cell membranes today is a silent metabolic fact that no blood panel in a standard physical examination reveals, that no standard cardiovascular risk assessment measures, and that no standard dietary guidance has yet succeeded in correcting at the population level. The experiment continues. The control group — the population eating traditional whole-food diets with ancestral fat ratios — is shrinking. The results are all around us.*

VIII. Questions Worth Asking

The omega-3 index — EPA plus DHA as a percentage of total red blood cell fatty acids — is the most validated biomarker of omega-3 status. An omega-3 index above eight percent is associated with the lowest cardiovascular risk; the average for Western populations is four to five percent. This is a simple, inexpensive blood test that measures the actual fatty acid composition of cell membranes — the most relevant indicator of whether the omega-3 intervention is reaching the cells that need it.

Plasma or RBC fatty acid profiles can also quantify the AA to EPA ratio (a direct measure of the eicosanoid-producing balance), the presence of oxidized lipid products suggesting ongoing lipid peroxidation, and the overall polyunsaturated to saturated ratio that predicts membrane oxidative stability. None of these measurements is on a standard clinical panel. All are available through specialized laboratories and represent genuinely actionable upstream information for individuals with cardiovascular disease risk, neurological symptoms, inflammatory conditions, or mood disorders.

The information in this chapter is educational and does not constitute clinical advice. Omega-3 supplementation at high doses may interact with anticoagulant medications and should be discussed with a physician in individuals on blood thinners. Fish oil quality varies significantly between products — third-party testing for oxidation and contaminant levels is advisable. The author does not offer clinical recommendations for any individual.

For the Clinically Curious

The Omega-3 Index — Validation and Cardiovascular Risk

The omega-3 index, defined as EPA + DHA as a percentage of total fatty acids in red blood cell membranes (standardized assay), was proposed by Harris and von Schacky in 2004 as a novel risk factor for sudden cardiac death. The index reflects dietary omega-3 intake integrated over the 120-day erythrocyte lifespan. An omega-3 index below 4% is associated with approximately ten-fold higher risk of sudden cardiac death compared to an index above 8%, based on prospective cohort data. The index is modifiable: EPA+DHA supplementation at 2-4g/day raises the omega-3 index by approximately 2-3 percentage points over 3-4 months. RBC fatty acid analysis (the omega-3 index assay) is available through multiple commercial laboratories and has begun to appear in cardiovascular risk stratification protocols in some clinical settings, though it remains far from standard practice.

4-Hydroxynonenal (4-HNE) — Mechanism of Seed Oil Toxicity

4-Hydroxynonenal is a major aldehyde product of linoleic acid oxidation during heating. It is formed when the C11 hydrogen of linoleic acid is abstracted by reactive oxygen species, initiating a lipid peroxidation chain that ultimately produces 4-HNE through beta-scission. 4-HNE is a potent Michael acceptor that forms covalent adducts with the cysteine, lysine, and histidine residues of proteins, impairing their function. At physiologically relevant concentrations (10-100 μM), 4-HNE impairs mitochondrial Complex I activity, induces ER stress, activates NF-κB, and modifies DNA. 4-HNE-protein adducts are measurable in human plasma and tissue, and are elevated in cardiovascular disease, neurodegeneration, and cancer. The concentrations of 4-HNE generated during cooking of polyunsaturated seed oils at typical frying temperatures (180-200°C) exceed these physiologically active concentrations in the oil itself. Saturated and monounsaturated fats generate dramatically less 4-HNE under the same conditions, providing a mechanistic basis for preferring these fats for high-temperature cooking.

REDUCE-IT — EPA vs. EPA+DHA Controversy

The REDUCE-IT trial (NEJM, 2018) randomized 8,179 statin-treated adults with elevated triglycerides and established cardiovascular disease or diabetes to icosapentaenoic acid ethyl ester (EPA only, 4g/day, Vascepa/Epanova) or mineral oil placebo, showing a 25% relative risk reduction in major cardiovascular events ($p<0.001$) at 4.9 years. The STRENGTH trial (JAMA, 2020) used a combination EPA+DHA product (omega-3 carboxylic acid, 4g/day) with corn oil placebo and showed no cardiovascular benefit. The divergent results have generated significant debate about whether the benefit in REDUCE-IT is attributable to EPA specifically, to the mineral oil placebo's adverse effects (which raised LDL and inflammatory markers), or to both. The EPA-only versus EPA+DHA distinction has not been definitively resolved, and the DHA-only evidence base is separate. The practical clinical message — that form, dose, and source of omega-3 supplementation matter — is clear even if the optimal specification remains contested.

Cluster 14

The Supporting Cast — Protective Compounds

The Phytonutrients, Carotenoids, Enzymes, Signaling Molecules, and Biological Inputs That Disappear When Food Is Processed and That Medicine Has Never Thought to Replace

> *"The Western diet did not merely fail to provide adequate vitamins and minerals. It eliminated entire categories of compounds that traditional foods had always contained — compounds whose absence medicine never thought to measure, whose roles it never thought to investigate, and whose loss it has never thought to name."*

I. The Invisible Elimination

Consider what Diana's plate looked like at sixty-two. A nutritional analysis of her diet would have found adequate protein, reasonable caloric intake, and a multivitamin she took each morning faithfully. What it would not have found — because no clinical nutrition assessment routinely asks these questions — was the near-complete absence of the compounds in this cluster. Her vegetables came from a can or a bag of frozen mixed greens. Her fruit intake was a glass of orange juice. Cruciferous vegetables appeared perhaps twice a month. Raw nuts, herbs, and spices were absent. She cooked exclusively with canola oil and used no traditional cooking fats. She had not eaten organ meats in forty years. She had never eaten fermented vegetables. Her gut had not encountered the bitter plant compounds that trigger digestive enzyme release since childhood.

Diana had begun losing central vision in her left eye three years earlier — age-related macular degeneration, her ophthalmologist said, monitoring it with annual retinal photographs. She had been managing polycystic ovary syndrome with metformin since her early thirties: insulin resistance, irregular cycles, and an androgen excess that nobody had ever connected to an inositol supply that her processed-food diet had never adequately provided. Eight years earlier her gallbladder had been removed, and since then, she had struggled with fatty-food intolerance that her gastroenterologist attributed to bile acid diarrhea and treated with cholestyramine — without once asking about the digestive enzyme cascade, the bile acid cycle, or the bromelain-free, papain-free, enzyme-depleted diet that had left her digestive infrastructure without its natural botanical supports. Three specialists. Three diagnoses. The crew behind the stage had been missing for decades, and no one in her clinical team had the framework to notice.

Nobody had told Diana that her diet had eliminated an entire class of biological inputs whose collective function — activating the body's own protective systems, providing tissue-specific antioxidant coverage, supporting digestion at its enzymatic foundation, modulating gene expression through hormetic pathways, and signaling to the circadian and cellular maintenance machinery — was not replaceable by any standard supplement or any standard dietary guideline. Because medicine had never named these functions as a category, their absence had never been identified as a problem. That is the purpose of this cluster.

II. The Crew Behind the Stage

Fifteen compounds make up the crew behind the stage — not musicians with assigned chairs in the orchestra, but the technical team without whom no performance is possible. They are not traditional nutrients in the sense that their absence produces a diagnosable deficiency syndrome. Their absence produces something subtler and more pervasive: a slow failure of the body's own protective and maintenance systems, whose consequences accumulate silently over decades before they become named conditions. They are organized here in five teams: The Signal Shapers (polyphenols), The Tissue Guardians (carotenoids), The Gateway Crew (digestive enzymes), The Signal Infrastructure (spermidine, inositol, and MSM), and The Lighting Department (light as biological input).

- **Sulforaphane** — the Nrf2 activator from cruciferous vegetables (broccoli, Brussels sprouts, kale, cabbage). The most potent known inducer of phase II detoxification enzymes. Absent from processed-food diets entirely.
- **Resveratrol** — from red grapes, berries, and peanuts. Activates SIRT1 and modulates mitochondrial biogenesis. Concentrated in foods that modern diets consume in diminished quantities.
- **Quercetin** — one of the most abundant flavonoids in food (onions, apples, capers). Anti-inflammatory, antiviral, and a zinc ionophore — it carries zinc into cells where it cannot enter unaided.

- **Curcumin** — from turmeric. NF-κB inhibitor, BDNF upregulator, and Nrf2 activator. Bioavailability is almost zero without piperine from black pepper and a fat vehicle — a preparation story that most supplementation ignores.
- **EGCG (epigallocatechin gallate)** — from green tea. Inhibits DNA methyltransferase (an epigenetic mechanism), modulates autophagy, and has documented cardiovascular and metabolic protective effects.
- **Anthocyanins** — from berries, purple sweet potato, black beans, red cabbage. Anti-inflammatory, vasodilatory, and associated with reduced cognitive decline risk in prospective studies.
- **Lutein and zeaxanthin** — carotenoids concentrated in the macula of the retina, where they absorb damaging blue light and provide the primary antioxidant defense against age-related macular degeneration. Found in eggs, kale, spinach, and corn.
- **Beta-carotene and lycopene** — carotenoids with tissue-specific antioxidant functions. Lycopene concentrates in the prostate and skin. Beta-carotene is a vitamin A precursor but has independent antioxidant roles in the lipid phase of cell membranes. Both are heat-released — cooking tomatoes and carrots increases bioavailability.
- **Bromelain and papain** — proteolytic enzymes from pineapple and papaya. Active at multiple pH ranges, anti-inflammatory, and capable of reducing circulating immune complexes when taken between meals. Among the few food-derived enzymes with documented systemic effects beyond the gut.
- **Nattokinase and serrapeptase** — microbial enzymes with fibrinolytic activity. Nattokinase, derived from the Japanese fermented soybean food natto, degrades fibrin and has documented effects on blood viscosity and cardiovascular risk markers. Serrapeptase, from silkworm gut bacteria, has anti-inflammatory and biofilm-disrupting properties with clinical evidence in sinusitis and venous insufficiency.

- **Spermidine** — a polyamine found in wheat germ, soybeans, aged cheese, and mushrooms. One of the most potent known dietary inducers of autophagy — the cellular self-cleaning process that clears damaged proteins, dysfunctional mitochondria, and intracellular debris. Spermidine intake from food is inversely associated with cardiovascular and all-cause mortality in prospective data.
- **Inositol** — a sugar alcohol found in fruits, beans, grains, and nuts, sometimes classified as a B vitamin (B8). A structural component of cell membranes as phosphatidylinositol, a second messenger in insulin signaling, and a compound with documented effects in PCOS, anxiety, and obsessive-compulsive spectrum conditions at therapeutic doses. Modern refined diets deliver substantially less than traditional whole-food diets.
- **MSM (methylsulfonylmethane)** — an organic sulfur compound found in fresh vegetables and fruits, destroyed by food processing. A bioavailable sulfur donor for glutathione synthesis, collagen formation, and joint cartilage integrity. The sulfur gap in processed-food diets is one of the least-discussed nutritional deficits in modern medicine.
- **I3C and DIM (indole-3-carbinol and diindolylmethane)** — compounds formed from glucosinolates in cruciferous vegetables during chewing and digestion. Modulate estrogen metabolism toward the less proliferative 2-hydroxyoestrone pathway, upregulate phase II detoxification, and have documented anti-cancer activity in cell and animal models. Absent from diets that do not include cruciferous vegetables.
- **Light as biological input** — not a nutrient in any classical sense, but a biological input whose withdrawal from modern indoor life produces measurable physiological consequences: reduced nitric oxide generation from skin UVB exposure, impaired cytochrome c oxidase stimulation by near-infrared wavelengths, and disrupted circadian entrainment. The human body evolved in sunlight. Its absence is a novel environmental condition whose biological consequences medicine has barely begun to characterize.

III. The Signal Shapers — Polyphenols and the Nrf2 Pathway

The Master Switch the Body Built for Plants

Plants do not have immune systems. They cannot run from environmental threats. Instead, they synthesize a vast pharmacopoeia of secondary metabolites — the polyphenols, flavonoids, glucosinolates, and terpenoids that give plants their colors, their bitterness, their pungency, and their resistance to pathogens and UV radiation. When humans eat these plants, they consume that pharmacopoeia. And the human body, shaped over millions of years of co-evolution with a plant-rich diet, has built dedicated receptor systems and signaling pathways for receiving and acting on these signals.

The most important of these signaling systems is the Nrf2 pathway. Nrf2 (nuclear factor erythroid 2-related factor 2) is a transcription factor — a protein that moves from the cytoplasm into the nucleus when activated, binds to antioxidant response elements (AREs) in DNA, and switches on the expression of over 200 protective genes. These include the phase II detoxification enzymes (glutathione S-transferases, quinone oxidoreductase, UDP-glucuronosyltransferases), the antioxidant enzymes (superoxide dismutase, catalase, glutathione peroxidase), heme oxygenase-1 (which degrades the pro-oxidant heme into the anti-inflammatory bilirubin), and the enzymes that synthesize glutathione itself.

Sulforaphane is the most potent dietary Nrf2 activator identified to date. It is formed when the enzyme myrosinase — released from cruciferous vegetable cells by chewing, chopping, or crushing — converts the glucosinolate glucoraphanin into sulforaphane. This is a plant defense mechanism that becomes, in the human gut, a powerful upregulator of the body's own antioxidant and detoxification machinery. A single serving of broccoli sprouts — which contain approximately fifty to one hundred times more glucoraphanin than mature broccoli — produces a sustained twelve-hour elevation of phase II enzyme activity. Clinical trials have demonstrated that sulforaphane-rich broccoli sprout extracts reduce oxidative stress markers in air-pollution-exposed populations, improve antioxidant enzyme activity in patients with type 2 diabetes, and exhibit anti-cancer activity in prostate epithelium.

Curcumin and resveratrol activate Nrf2 by different mechanisms but produce overlapping effects: increased glutathione synthesis, upregulation of antioxidant enzymes, and suppression of NF-κB — the parallel transcription factor that drives pro-inflammatory gene expression. NF-κB and Nrf2 exist in a reciprocal relationship: when NF-κB is high, Nrf2 tends to be low, and the inflammatory and oxidative burden compounds. Polyphenols that simultaneously activate Nrf2 and suppress NF-κB are performing a dual function that no pharmaceutical anti-inflammatory currently replicates in its entirety.

Quercetin as Zinc Ionophore — A Cross-Cluster Connection

Quercetin's role as a zinc ionophore illustrates why polyphenols cannot be understood in isolation from the mineral environment in which they operate. Zinc is essential for antiviral defense — it inhibits RNA-dependent RNA polymerase, the enzyme coronaviruses and influenza viruses use to replicate their genomes. But zinc cannot cross cell membranes unaided. It requires a transport mechanism. Quercetin acts as that mechanism, chelating zinc and carrying it across the lipid bilayer into the cytoplasm where it can inhibit viral replication. In conditions of zinc adequacy but quercetin absence — the typical processed-food dietary situation — the zinc is present but cannot reach its intracellular target at the concentrations required for antiviral activity. This is a nutritional synergy that no single-nutrient analysis would ever reveal.

IV. The Tissue Guardians — Carotenoids and Tissue-Specific Protection

Why the Macula Requires Its Own Antioxidants

The macula — the central region of the retina responsible for high-acuity vision — is one of the metabolically most active tissues in the human body. It is continuously exposed to blue-wavelength light, which generates reactive oxygen species in the retinal pigment epithelium with each photon absorbed. The tissue's defense against this sustained oxidative challenge is the macular pigment: a dense deposit of lutein and zeaxanthin, two carotenoids that absorb blue light before it reaches the photoreceptors and quench the reactive oxygen species generated by light exposure. Macular pigment optical density — a direct measure of lutein and zeaxanthin accumulation in the retina — is the single most modifiable risk factor for age-related macular degeneration that exists.

The AREDS2 trial — the Age-Related Eye Disease Study 2, funded by the National Eye Institute — demonstrated that supplementation with lutein (10 mg/day) and zeaxanthin (2 mg/day), combined with vitamins C and E, zinc, and copper, reduced the risk of progression from intermediate to advanced macular degeneration by twenty-five percent over five years. Lutein and zeaxanthin are found in egg yolks, kale, spinach, and corn. A diet that avoids egg yolks on cardiovascular grounds and consumes minimal dark leafy greens is systematically depleting the macula's primary defense against the most common cause of irreversible vision loss in adults over sixty. This is not a theoretical risk. It is a quantifiable dietary exposure that conventional ophthalmology almost never assesses.

Lycopene concentrates in a different tissue: the prostate, and the skin. The prostate accumulates lycopene from dietary sources — predominantly cooked tomatoes and tomato products — at concentrations substantially higher than plasma levels. Epidemiological studies consistently find that higher lycopene intake is associated with reduced prostate cancer risk, and mechanistic studies confirm lycopene's ability to inhibit androgen receptor signaling and induce apoptosis in prostate epithelial cells. The cooking requirement matters: lycopene in raw tomatoes is bound in a geometric configuration (all-trans) that has poor bioavailability. Cooking converts it to cis-lycopene, which is substantially better absorbed and is the form that accumulates in prostate tissue. The prostate is protected not by the raw tomato but by the cooked one — a nutritional fact that processed-food diets supplying sauce from a can happen to provide, while fresh-food diets that serve raw salad do not.

V. The Gateway Crew — Digestive Enzymes and the Forgotten Foundation

When Digestion Starts to Fail Quietly

Every nutrient discussed in this book must first be liberated from food by digestive enzymes before it can be absorbed. Protein requires protease activity to be cleaved into the amino acids that Cluster 11 describes. Carbohydrates require amylase. Fats require lipase, and the bile acids whose synthesis depends on the liver's cholesterol metabolism. Fat-soluble vitamins — A, D, E, K — require bile for micellar solubilization before absorption. The mineral absorption mechanisms of Cluster 13 depend on stomach acid and the reducing conditions it creates. The entire upstream nutrient supply to every cluster is mediated through digestive capacity that declines with age, worsens with acid-suppressive medications, and is rarely directly assessed.

Gastric acid secretion declines with age (hypochlorhydria), with chronic proton pump inhibitor use, and with H. pylori infection. Pancreatic enzyme secretion declines in parallel. The consequence is a systematic impairment of protein digestion that presents as bloating, early satiety, and food sensitivities rather than as a named deficiency — a pattern that medicine attributes to irritable bowel syndrome or functional dyspepsia and addresses with antispasmodics rather than digestive support. The nutrients that fail to be absorbed — zinc, iron, B12, magnesium, the fat-soluble vitamins — produce downstream deficiencies in every cluster, but the upstream digestive failure that created them is rarely the target of clinical intervention.

Bromelain and papain are plant-derived proteases active across a broader pH range than pancreatic enzymes, which makes them functional in the acidic stomach environment where pancreatic proteases cannot operate. Taken with meals, they supplement the body's own protein-digesting capacity. Taken between meals on an empty stomach, they enter the bloodstream to a small extent and exert systemic anti-inflammatory effects — reducing circulating immune complexes and inflammatory mediators — that have been documented in randomized trials for post-surgical recovery, osteoarthritis, and sinusitis. Bromelain has also demonstrated fibrinolytic properties, reducing platelet aggregation and thinning blood in a manner that has prompted investigation in cardiovascular risk reduction.

Nattokinase — a serine protease from Bacillus subtilis var. natto — has a more targeted mechanism: it directly degrades fibrin, the protein scaffold of blood clots, and has shown documented reductions in fibrinogen and D-dimer levels in clinical trials. An estimated twelve million Japanese people consume natto regularly, a dietary pattern associated with lower cardiovascular mortality in that population. Whether the cardiovascular protection attributed to Japanese diet is partly mediated by nattokinase rather than by fish consumption alone is an unresolved question that Western clinical nutrition has shown limited interest in pursuing. Nattokinase supplements are available and have a reasonable safety profile at standard doses, with the expected precaution for anticoagulated patients.

VI. The Signal Infrastructure — Spermidine, Inositol, MSM, and the Overlooked Trio

Autophagy, Second Messengers, and the Sulfur Gap

Spermidine is named after its first identification in semen, though it is ubiquitous in living cells — present in wheat germ, soybeans, aged cheese, mushrooms, peas, and corn. It is a naturally occurring polyamine whose intracellular concentration declines with age in parallel with declining autophagy capacity. Autophagy — the process by which cells enclose damaged organelles, misfolded proteins, and intracellular pathogens in autophagosomes and deliver them to lysosomes for digestion — is one of the body's primary mechanisms for cellular maintenance, healthy aging, and cancer prevention. When autophagy declines, misfolded proteins accumulate (a hallmark of neurodegeneration), dysfunctional mitochondria persist (reducing cellular energy and increasing reactive oxygen species), and senescent cells resist the clearance that normally follows cellular damage.

A prospective cohort study from Vienna following over 800 participants for twenty years found that dietary spermidine intake was inversely associated with all-cause mortality in a dose-dependent manner, with the highest quintile of intake associated with a five-year difference in life expectancy compared to the lowest. The mechanism is primarily autophagy induction via inhibition of EP300 (a histone acetyltransferase), which mimics the effects of caloric restriction at the cellular signaling level. Spermidine, in this framing, is not a supplement. It is a dietary signal that the body's cellular maintenance machinery has been listening for throughout evolutionary time — a signal that processed-food diets no longer reliably deliver.

Inositol occupies a different mechanistic territory. As phosphatidylinositol, it is a structural membrane component that serves as the substrate for the phosphoinositide signaling pathway — one of the major second messenger systems through which insulin, growth factors, and neurotransmitter receptors communicate with the cell interior. Inositol hexaphosphate (IP6) is the storage form of phosphorus in plant seeds and is a ligand for multiple signaling proteins. Clinical evidence has accumulated for myo-inositol (one of the nine stereoisomers) in polycystic ovary syndrome, where doses of 2–4 g/day improve insulin sensitivity, restore menstrual regularity, and reduce androgen levels in randomized trials; and for the combination of myo-inositol and D-chiro-inositol in gestational diabetes risk reduction. Inositol at higher doses (12–18 g/day) has been studied in panic disorder and obsessive-compulsive disorder, where it has shown effects comparable to SSRIs in small trials — a finding that remains underutilized in psychiatric practice.

MSM — methylsulfonylmethane — is the dietary sulfur compound that receives least clinical attention despite being one of the most widely consumed supplements globally. It is formed in the atmosphere from oceanic dimethyl sulfide and enters the food chain through plants, concentrating in fresh vegetables, fruit, meat, and milk. Food processing — particularly heating and pasteurization — destroys MSM. The consequence is a systematic reduction in bioavailable organic sulfur in processed-food diets that is not compensated by inorganic sulfate. MSM provides sulfur for glutathione synthesis (supplementing the cysteine pathway of Cluster 4), for collagen cross-linking (supplementing the structural network of Cluster 5), and for cartilage proteoglycan synthesis. Randomized trials in osteoarthritis have consistently shown MSM supplementation (1.5–3 g/day) reduces pain and improves joint function, with a safety profile comparable to placebo. The sulfur gap in modern diets is real, measurable, and addressable — and it receives almost no clinical attention.

VII. I3C, DIM, and Hormonal Detoxification

Indole-3-carbinol (I3C) is formed when glucobrassicin — a glucosinolate concentrated in cruciferous vegetables — is hydrolyzed by myrosinase during chewing and digestion. In the acidic stomach environment, I3C undergoes further condensation to form diindolylmethane (DIM), the compound primarily responsible for the estrogen-modulating effects attributed to cruciferous vegetable consumption. DIM shifts estrogen metabolism toward the 2-hydroxyoestrone pathway — a less biologically active metabolite that does not stimulate estrogen-receptor-positive cell proliferation — and away from the 16α-hydroxyoestrone and 4-hydroxyoestrone pathways associated with carcinogenic activity in breast tissue. This metabolic shift is measurable in urine by the 2:16 hydroxyoestrone ratio, a biomarker that several integrative medicine practitioners use to assess breast cancer risk — and that conventional oncology almost never orders.

DIM also upregulates phase II detoxification enzymes through Nrf2 activation, connects to the methylation network through its influence on the COMT enzyme (catechol-O-methyltransferase) that inactivates catechol estrogens, and interacts with the aryl hydrocarbon receptor (AhR) — a transcription factor that regulates immune cell differentiation, particularly the balance between regulatory T cells and Th17 inflammatory cells. The compounds in cruciferous vegetables, in other words, are not simply antioxidants. They are modulators of hormonal clearance, immune balance, and gene expression that operate at multiple levels simultaneously. A diet that excludes cruciferous vegetables is not merely lower in certain vitamins. It has lost an entire set of hormonal and immunological signaling inputs.

VIII. The Lighting Department — Light as Biological Input

The Spectrum Medicine Has Not Considered

Homo sapiens evolved under full-spectrum sunlight for approximately three hundred thousand years. We spent our days outdoors, with light exposure that varied across the full solar spectrum — ultraviolet, visible, and near-infrared — in a pattern synchronized to the solar day. For the last century, and with accelerating intensity in the last four decades, we have moved that existence indoors. Modern office workers may spend ninety-five percent of their waking hours under artificial lighting that delivers blue-spectrum visible light but virtually none of the UVB, near-infrared, or full-spectrum visible light that characterized the evolutionary environment. This is not a minor modification to lifestyle. It is a fundamental change in the biological inputs the human body receives, one whose consequences medicine has barely begun to characterize.

The most established consequence is vitamin D synthesis — the UVB-driven conversion of 7-dehydrocholesterol in skin to previtamin D3, covered in detail in Cluster 12. But sunlight has biological effects that are entirely independent of vitamin D. UVB radiation striking the skin causes the release of nitric oxide from nitrite and nitroso compounds stored in the epidermis — a mechanism that lowers blood pressure by vasodilating peripheral blood vessels. Studies exposing subjects to simulated sunlight demonstrate blood pressure reductions of several mmHg within minutes of exposure, an effect that vitamin D supplementation alone does not replicate. The dose of UVB required is sub-erythemic — below the threshold that causes sunburn — and represents the kind of regular, modest sun exposure that characterized outdoor existence for essentially the entire history of the human species.

Near-infrared light — wavelengths from approximately 700 to 1100 nanometres — is absorbed by cytochrome c oxidase, the terminal enzyme of the mitochondrial electron transport chain and the same enzyme discussed in Cluster 1 in the context of copper and cellular energy production. Near-infrared photons increase cytochrome c oxidase activity, accelerating electron transfer and increasing ATP production. In tissues with mitochondrial dysfunction — aging neurons, metabolically stressed cardiac tissue, inflamed joints — near-infrared light has demonstrated therapeutic effects in a growing body of clinical evidence. Photobiomodulation, the clinical application of specific light wavelengths to biological tissue, is an active research field with over five hundred published randomized trials. It remains almost entirely outside mainstream clinical practice. The sun, which has always delivered near-infrared as part of its full-spectrum output, was providing this photobiomodulation stimulus to outdoor human populations continuously throughout evolutionary history. It is now absent for most people most of the time.

Circadian light entrainment represents the third major axis. The suprachiasmatic nucleus — the master clock of the circadian system — receives its primary timing signal from blue-wavelength light detected by intrinsically photosensitive retinal ganglion cells containing the photopigment melanopsin. Morning bright light exposure entrains the circadian pacemaker to solar time, sets the timing of cortisol awakening response, and calibrates the rhythms of sleep, digestion, immune function, and cellular repair that the entire body follows. Chronic disruption of circadian entrainment — through insufficient morning light, excessive evening blue light from screens, and irregular sleep timing — is associated with metabolic syndrome, impaired immune function, elevated inflammatory markers, and accelerated aging at the cellular level. This is not a speculative connection. The circadian biology of the last three decades has produced one of the most mechanistically detailed accounts in all of chronobiology, recognized by the 2017 Nobel Prize in Physiology or Medicine.

IX. The Web of Dependencies

Sulforaphane connects to Cluster 10: Nrf2 activation by sulforaphane is the primary dietary mechanism for upregulating the phase II enzymes that make detoxification possible. A diet absent of cruciferous vegetables is a diet with systematically impaired phase II capacity, regardless of how well the liver is otherwise supported.

Quercetin connects to Cluster 8: As a zinc ionophore, quercetin determines whether the zinc available from dietary or supplemental sources reaches its intracellular targets in immune cells. Zinc adequacy without quercetin is zinc that cannot fully execute its antiviral role.

Resveratrol connects to Cluster 1: SIRT1 activation by resveratrol stimulates mitochondrial biogenesis through PGC-1α, the same pathway activated by PQQ and NAD+ precursors. These compounds converge on the same mitochondrial maintenance program from different entry points.

MSM connects to Cluster 4 and Cluster 5: Sulfur from MSM feeds into the cysteine pathway for glutathione synthesis (Cluster 4) and into the structural requirements for collagen cross-linking (Cluster 5). Sulfur deficiency impairs both simultaneously.

Light connects to Cluster 1 and Cluster 6: Near-infrared stimulation of cytochrome c oxidase directly augments mitochondrial ATP production (Cluster 1). Circadian entrainment by morning light governs the cortisol awakening response and the timing of thyroid hormone cycling (Cluster 6). Light is not separate from biochemistry. It is an input into it.

Inositol connects to Cluster 9: Phosphatidylinositol synthesis requires choline (Cluster 9's phospholipid context), and inositol's role in insulin signaling intersects with the metabolic methylation demands discussed in that cluster. The membrane signaling system and the methylation system are not independent.

X. Questions Worth Asking

No standard clinical laboratory panel measures lutein and zeaxanthin status, despite the existence of a validated device (macular pigment optical density, or MPOD) that quantifies these carotenoids non-invasively in the retina in under five minutes. No standard clinical encounter asks about cruciferous vegetable consumption, despite the documented relationship between I3C/DIM exposure and estrogen metabolism pathways that determine breast cancer risk. No standard nutrition assessment asks about spermidine intake, despite prospective evidence that dietary spermidine is one of the strongest food-derived predictors of longevity in the available data. No standard metabolic workup includes inositol status, despite clinical trial evidence for its utility in PCOS and gestational diabetes that would justify a question about it in any woman presenting with insulin resistance. And no standard clinical history asks how much time a patient spends outdoors, despite the documented consequences of sunlight deprivation on nitric oxide generation, circadian function, and cytochrome c oxidase activity.

What would it mean to take these questions seriously? It would mean recognizing that the Western diet has not merely created deficiencies in the classical nutrients — the vitamins, the minerals, the essential fatty acids — that the other thirteen clusters describe. It has also eliminated an entire category of protective biological inputs whose collective function — activating phase II enzymes, protecting tissue-specific antioxidant reserves, supporting digestive capacity, inducing autophagy, modulating hormonal clearance, and signaling to the circadian and mitochondrial maintenance machinery — was never designed to be replaceable by a multivitamin. These inputs were always provided by diet. Diet has stopped providing them. Medicine has not noticed, because medicine was never looking for them.

Diana's macular degeneration was not inevitable. Her PCOS was not simply hormonal bad luck. Her digestive struggle after gallbladder removal was not simply a surgical consequence to be managed indefinitely with a binding resin. They were the accumulated consequence of a diet that had quietly eliminated an entire category of biological inputs that her body had always been designed to receive. The question is not whether these compounds matter. The question is whether anyone thought to ask whether they were present.

The information in this chapter is educational and does not constitute clinical advice. Several compounds described here — including bromelain, nattokinase, and serrapeptase — have anticoagulant or fibrinolytic properties and should be discussed with a physician before use in individuals taking anticoagulant or antiplatelet medications. I3C and DIM modulate cytochrome P450 enzyme activity and may affect the metabolism of medications processed through these pathways. Inositol at high doses should be discussed with a physician in pregnancy. The author does not offer clinical recommendations for any individual.

For the Clinically Curious

Nrf2 — The Antioxidant Response Element and Hormetic Activation

Nrf2 is held in the cytoplasm by its inhibitor protein Keap1 under basal conditions. Keap1 acts as a sensor for electrophilic and oxidative stress: when electrophilic compounds — including sulforaphane, curcumin, and resveratrol — modify cysteine residues on Keap1, the Keap1-Nrf2 complex dissociates. Free Nrf2 translocates to the nucleus, dimerises with small Maf proteins, and binds antioxidant response elements (AREs) in the promoter regions of over 200 cytoprotective genes. This is a hormetic mechanism: a low-level stressor (the electrophilic plant compound) triggers an adaptive protective response that is disproportionately larger than the stress itself. The biological rationale for consuming bitter, pungent, and colorful plant compounds is not that they contain antioxidants directly — most polyphenols have limited direct antioxidant capacity in vivo — but that they activate the body's own antioxidant gene expression program, which operates at far greater scale and specificity than any exogenous antioxidant supplement could achieve.

Lutein and Zeaxanthin — Macular Pigment Optical Density and the AREDS2 Evidence

Macular pigment optical density (MPOD) is measured by

heterochromatic flicker photometry — a non-invasive psychophysical test that takes approximately five minutes. MPOD has been validated against post-mortem macular carotenoid concentration and correlates with dietary lutein and zeaxanthin intake. The AREDS2 trial (n=4,203, five-year follow-up, NEJM 2013) demonstrated that substituting beta-carotene in the original AREDS formula with lutein (10 mg/day) and zeaxanthin (2 mg/day) reduced the risk of progression to advanced AMD by 26% compared to no lutein/zeaxanthin, and by 18% compared to the original AREDS formula including beta-carotene. Crucially, the reduction in risk was greatest in participants in the lowest quintile of dietary lutein and zeaxanthin intake at baseline — confirming that the effect is nutritional replacement of an inadequate dietary supply rather than pharmacological supplementation above adequate levels. MPOD measurement is available in optometry practices equipped with heterochromatic flicker photometers and represents one of the few non-invasive nutritional biomarkers with direct tissue-level validity and therapeutic implications.

Spermidine and Autophagy — EP300 Inhibition and the Caloric Restriction Mimetic

Spermidine induces autophagy primarily through inhibition of EP300, a histone acetyltransferase that acetylates proteins including Atg proteins (autophagy-related proteins) required for autophagosome formation. EP300 inhibition by spermidine hypoacetylates Atg proteins, activating them and initiating the autophagy cascade. This mechanism is independent of the mTOR and AMPK pathways through which caloric restriction and rapamycin induce autophagy — making spermidine a complementary rather than redundant autophagy inducer. The Graz Longitudinal Study of Mental Health and Aging (LONGEVITY, n=829, 20-year follow-up) found that higher dietary spermidine intake was associated with lower all-cause mortality (HR 0.60, 95% CI 0.37–0.96 for highest versus lowest quartile) and with lower cardiovascular mortality specifically. Wheat germ contains the highest concentrations of spermidine in common foods (~243 nmol/g), followed by soybeans and aged cheese. Modern refined flour — which removes the wheat germ — delivers essentially none.

The Orchestra in Full

What Happens When All Fourteen Clusters Play Together — and What Margaret Deserved

"A physician who knows only one nutrient is less dangerous than a physician who knows none — but only barely. The body is not a collection of nutrient stories. It is a single story, told in sixty languages simultaneously."

I. The Night Margaret's Orchestra Played

Picture Margaret at fifty-three — the same woman we met in the opening pages. Hypertension. Hypothyroidism. Generalized anxiety. A chronic skin condition. Unexplained fatigue for three years. Bleeding gums. Borderline cholesterol. Five physicians. Five medications. Three to five thousand dollars per year. No answers.

Now picture the orchestra behind her symptoms. Not five separate diseases requiring five separate specialists. One orchestra, playing poorly in fourteen sections simultaneously, each section's underperformance compounding the others, the sound that reached the clinical ear so degraded by the time it emerged as a named condition that the upstream music was completely unrecognizable.

Her energy architecture (Cluster 1) was impaired: magnesium insufficiency reducing ATP activation, thiamine demand elevated by years of chronic stress and a carbohydrate-heavy diet, CoQ10 potentially depleted by the beta-blocker that had been prescribed for her hypertension, copper in question given her never-measured zinc-copper ratio. Her gut gateway (Cluster 2) was compromised: three years on a proton pump inhibitor impeding mineral absorption, four antibiotic courses disrupting the microbiome whose restoration was never addressed, a processed-food diet providing emulsifiers that damaged her mucus layer while delivering insufficient prebiotic fiber. Her microbiome (Cluster 3) had been repeatedly devastated and never rebuilt: butyrate production likely insufficient, tryptophan diversion toward kynurenine rather than serotonin — contributing to her anxiety and mood — enhanced by the LPS-mediated neuroinflammation that leaked through her damaged gut wall.

Her antioxidant shield (Cluster 4) had gaps: selenium never measured, glutathione status unknown, the oxidative stress of chronic inflammation and medication metabolism creating demand that her unassessed network may not have been meeting. Her structural architecture (Cluster 5) was visibly failing at her gums — the bleeding that dentistry attributed to poor flossing technique was a systemic collagen integrity failure requiring ascorbate, copper, and glycine, none of which had been addressed. Her hormonal regulators (Cluster 6) included a thyroid axis that her medication replaced at the hormone level while leaving five upstream nutrient dependencies — selenium, zinc, iron, iodine, vitamin A — entirely unaddressed, and an insulin system stressed by a decade of magnesium depletion. Her neurological foundations (Cluster 7) were operating on depleted B vitamins and an omega-3 profile unknown to anyone in her care team, producing the anxiety that her SSRI was partly managing and the cognitive fog that she had stopped mentioning because nobody had ever acted on it.

Her immune architects (Cluster 8) were miscalibrated by vitamin D insufficiency — one low-normal result, a supplement recommendation that may not have been followed up — and by the gut dysbiosis that was providing impaired regulatory T-cell education. Her methylation network (Cluster 9) had never been assessed: homocysteine unmeasured, MTHFR status unknown, the folate-B12-riboflavin triad that drives methylation and determines her capacity for neurotransmitter regulation, gene expression, and cardiovascular risk never optimized. Her detoxification network (Cluster 10) was processing five medications continuously, with phase II conjugation capacity that nobody had ever considered. Her amino acid foundation (Cluster 11) included glycine that her collagen-poor diet was not providing and glutamine that her damaged gut was consuming at rates her diet was not replacing. Her fat-soluble foundations (Cluster 12) included vitamin D insufficiency that was documented and inadequately addressed, vitamin K2 that was absent from her processed-food diet, and vitamin A status that nobody had thought to connect to her recurring skin condition and her impaired mucosal immunity. And the fatty acid ratio in her cell membranes (Cluster 13) — shaped by years of seed-oil-heavy processed food and minimal fatty fish consumption — was producing the elevated inflammatory baseline that was driving her cardiovascular risk and contributing to her neurological and immune dysregulation. The supporting cast (Cluster 14) was almost entirely absent: no cruciferous vegetables, no dietary spermidine, no quercetin-containing foods in meaningful quantities, no lutein-rich eggs or dark greens, no time outdoors, and a diet wholly devoid of the phytonutrients whose collective function — activating her phase II enzymes, protecting her macular pigment, inducing autophagy, and modulating her estrogen metabolism — medicine had never thought to assess.

Fourteen sections. Every one of them impaired. Every one of them impacting the others. The sound that emerged — labeled hypertension, hypothyroidism, anxiety, a skin condition, unexplained fatigue, and bleeding gums — was the noise of an orchestra trying to perform on an empty stage with missing instruments, depleted musicians, and a concert hall that had not been maintained for years.

II. The Interactions Medicine Missed

How the Clusters Compound Each Other

Reading this book cluster by cluster reveals each section of the orchestra separately. But the most important phenomenon in nutritional medicine is not what happens in each section individually — it is what happens when multiple sections are impaired simultaneously. The consequences are not additive. They are multiplicative. Each insufficiency creates demand that the depleted adjacent system cannot meet, and the failure cascades.

When the gut gateway fails (Cluster 2), every other cluster is affected — because every nutrient that feeds every other system must first pass through that gateway. The energy architects (Cluster 1) receive fewer minerals. The antioxidant shield (Cluster 4) receives less selenium and zinc. The neurological foundations (Cluster 7) receive less B12 and less of the iron that tryptophan hydroxylase requires to produce serotonin. The structural architects (Cluster 5) receive less copper for lysyl oxidase and less vitamin C for prolyl hydroxylase. When the gut fails first, every subsequent nutritional intervention is limited by the efficiency of the gateway through which it must pass.

When the methylation network (Cluster 9) is impaired, the detoxification network (Cluster 10) loses its primary methylation pathway for estrogen and catecholamine inactivation, increasing the liver's burden on alternative pathways. The neurological foundations (Cluster 7) lose their SAMe supply for neurotransmitter regulation. The antioxidant shield (Cluster 4) loses glutathione production because cysteine flow through the transsulfuration pathway is impaired when homocysteine is not being efficiently recycled. One methylation impairment touches four clusters simultaneously.

When the essential fatty acid ratio is skewed toward omega-6 (Cluster 13), every cell membrane in every organ becomes more inflammatory in its basal signaling tone. The immune architects (Cluster 8) produce more pro-inflammatory eicosanoids and fewer resolution mediators. The neurological foundations (Cluster 7) operate in neuronal membranes that are less fluid and less efficient. The structural architects (Cluster 5) work on a collagen matrix that is surrounded by a more inflamed extracellular environment. The gut gateway (Cluster 2) operates in a mucosal immune milieu that is more likely to mount inappropriate inflammatory responses. One fatty acid imbalance touches every cluster.

When the supporting cast is absent (Cluster 14), the body's own protective gene expression program goes unstimulated. The Nrf2 pathway — which governs over 200 cytoprotective genes including the phase II detoxification enzymes that the detoxification network (Cluster 10) requires to conjugate medication metabolites, the antioxidant enzymes that the antioxidant shield (Cluster 4) depends on for regeneration, and the glutathione synthesis enzymes that feed every cluster that uses glutathione as a cofactor — operates at basal rather than induced levels. Macular pigment optical density declines in the retina as lutein and zeaxanthin are not replaced. Autophagy slows as spermidine is removed from the dietary supply. Estrogen metabolism shifts toward the proliferative 16α pathway as I3C and DIM disappear with cruciferous vegetables. Circadian entrainment degrades as indoor life eliminates the morning light signal the suprachiasmatic nucleus was designed to receive. One category of biological input, absent from the diet, simultaneously impairs detoxification capacity, visual protection, cellular maintenance, hormonal clearance, and circadian function. No standard clinical assessment notices any of it.

III. The Triage Hierarchy

When multiple clusters are simultaneously insufficient, the body does not fail in all of them equally. It triages. Bruce Ames's triage theory — one of the most important conceptual frameworks in nutritional science — predicts that when micronutrients are scarce, the body allocates them first to functions that support immediate survival at the expense of functions that protect long-term health.

ATP production is prioritized over antioxidant defense. Immune activation is prioritized over immune regulation. Tissue repair is prioritized over long-term structural maintenance. Neurotransmitter production is prioritized over neuronal protection. The triage keeps the person alive and functional in the short term. Over years and decades, however, the functions that have been downregulated accumulate their deficits: the antioxidant defense gaps lead to oxidative damage in arterial walls and neuronal DNA; the immune regulation gaps allow autoimmune sensitization to develop; the structural maintenance gap allows the collagen architecture to slowly degrade; the neuronal protection gap allows the mitochondrial DNA mutations that accumulate with inadequately defended oxidative stress to progressively impair neurological function.

This triage model explains something that has puzzled nutritional medicine: why the consequences of micronutrient insufficiency so often emerge decades after the insufficiency begins. The person does not immediately develop the condition that the insufficiency will eventually cause. They develop subtle functional impairments — slower recovery, reduced resilience, gradually declining performance — that represent the triage operating as designed. The disease emerges when the triage-deferred deficits reach the threshold of clinical visibility. By that point, years or decades of upstream causes have accumulated.

Ames described the triage — how a body short on micronutrients spends them. The *Invisible Famine Hypothesis*, set out at the opening of this book, describes *why* a body surrounded by modern food enters triage at all. The nutrient sensors that evolved over two million years cannot distinguish a failed harvest from a full plate stripped of its nourishment; both read as scarcity, and scarcity activates the ancient response. Margaret's fourteen clusters are not fourteen separate failures. They are the switches that response turned off, one section of the orchestra at a time — powered down not because her body was broken, but because it was doing exactly what it was built to do in a famine it had no way of knowing was invisible.

IV. Margaret's Children: Triage Timeline Accelerating

Margaret was fifty-three when the orchestra's failure finally became loud enough for medicine to name. Her children do not have that long.

The triage model described in the preceding section was calibrated on a generation that began with reasonable nutritional reserves and depleted them gradually over decades under moderate stress. The consequences emerged in midlife — the hypertension, the hypothyroidism, the unexplained fatigue, the bleeding gums — because that is how long it took the deferred maintenance deficits to reach the threshold of clinical visibility. That timeline assumed a starting point of reasonable adequacy. It assumed a stress burden that, while real, was not the chronic, cortisol-saturating, nutrient-consuming load that defines daily life for the generation now in their twenties and thirties. And it assumed a food supply that, however imperfect, was less depleted than the one that generation inherited.

None of those assumptions hold anymore.

Margaret's children were formed in utero by mothers whose own nutritional status was already compromised by a more processed food supply than the generation before them. They were shaped in childhood by antibiotic courses whose consequences for microbiome diversity and immune education persisted for years without restoration. They grew up indoors, under artificial light, deprived of the outdoor bright-light exposure that triggers retinal dopamine release and inhibits the axial elongation of the developing eye — producing the myopia epidemic now affecting the majority of urban young adults at rates that one generation ago would have been considered extraordinary. They entered adulthood carrying stress burdens — chronic, cortisol-elevating, magnesium-consuming, thiamine-depleting — that accelerate nutrient depletion at rates the original triage model never anticipated. They are running the triage algorithm starting further from adequacy, under greater demand, with fewer reserves, than any previous generation in the modern era.

The consequences are no longer arriving in decades. They are arriving in years — and they are arriving with a recognizable face that clinicians are seeing with increasing frequency without yet assembling into a pattern.

Cardiovascular risk markers — elevated homocysteine, impaired endothelial function, early arterial stiffness — are now documented in people in their twenties, in populations eating the diets that modern food guidelines consider adequate. Anxiety and depression are presenting in teenagers at rates that would have been unrecognizable a generation ago, and responding to first-line pharmaceutical treatment at rates that suggest the upstream nutritional substrate is not being addressed — the serotonin that requires iron and B6 to synthesize, the dopamine that requires iron, B6, copper, and vitamin C in sequence, the GABA that requires B6 to be converted from glutamate, the neuronal membrane architecture that requires DHA to transmit every signal efficiently. The medication is acting on a system whose raw materials were never assessed.

ADHD diagnoses have risen in lockstep with the dietary changes this book describes, and the nutritional substrate of the dopaminergic system that ADHD implicates has rarely been the subject of clinical investigation before the prescription pad is reached. Iron — the rate-limiting cofactor for tyrosine hydroxylase, the enzyme that produces dopamine — is consistently low in ADHD populations across multiple studies. Zinc, which modulates dopamine transporter activity and predicts stimulant medication response, is routinely unmeasured. Magnesium deficiency produces the hyperexcitability and distractibility that overlaps significantly with ADHD presentation. Omega-3 DHA — the structural fat of the prefrontal cortex, the seat of executive function and impulse control — is insufficient in the diets of most children presenting with attention difficulties. The question this book is positioned to ask is not whether ADHD is real. It is whether the upstream nutritional substrate of the developing dopamine system was ever assessed before the diagnosis was confirmed and the stimulant prescribed. In most clinical encounters, it was not. It was not because nobody was trained to ask, not because the question was considered and rejected.

The pattern extends further than the conditions already named. Chronic fatigue following viral illness — the mitochondrial substrate of Cluster 1 exposed by a stressor the depleted system could not absorb — is among the most common and most dismissed complaints in people under thirty-five, and the post-COVID era has made its nutritional substrate impossible to ignore. The gut disorder epidemic is the antibiotic legacy made visible: the twenty-five-year-old with IBS, multiplying food sensitivities, and a microbiome that repeated childhood antibiotic courses depleted and no subsequent intervention rebuilt. Autoimmune conditions — Hashimoto's, psoriasis, rheumatoid arthritis — are rising in prevalence and falling in age of onset, driven by the same barrier failure and vitamin D, selenium, and zinc insufficiency that Clusters 2 and 8 describe. Margaret has Hashimoto's at fifty-three. Her children are developing it at twenty-eight.

The hormonal and dermatological picture completes the pattern. PCOS affecting one in eight young women, managed with metformin without assessment of inositol, I3C, or omega-6 driven prostaglandin excess. Endometriosis dismissed for an average of seven years before diagnosis, its inflammatory substrate never connected to the fatty acid ratio of Cluster 13. Acne treated with antibiotics or isotretinoin — a synthetic vitamin A derivative — without checking zinc, omega-3 index, or gut barrier integrity. Eczema rising in children whose atopic immune skewing reflects the same dysbiosis and vitamin D insufficiency that the gut and immune clusters describe. Each of these is a triage signal. Each is being treated at the surface. None of the upstream questions are being asked.

Premature graying — once attributed to genetics and stress in vague terms — is appearing in the mid-twenties with a mechanistic precision that the triage model predicts exactly. Copper insufficiency impairs tyrosinase, the enzyme that converts tyrosine to melanin. Hydrogen peroxide accumulates in the hair follicle when antioxidant capacity is inadequate, bleaching pigment from within. Noradrenaline released during chronic stress depletes melanocyte stem cells from the follicle at an accelerated rate — a mechanism confirmed in landmark research that made the connection between the stress response and graying biologically precise rather than merely intuitive. Triage written in the hair, visible to anyone who looks, connected to the nutrient clusters in this book by mechanisms that are not speculative but documented.

Premature skin aging reflects the same collagen insufficiency that produces Margaret's bleeding gums, arriving earlier because the structural substrate — the vitamin C, copper, glycine, and zinc that build and cross-link collagen — was thinner to begin with and has been depleted faster. Fertility is declining across both sexes at timelines that epidemiologists are struggling to fully explain, and that the zinc, selenium, CoQ10, and omega-3 dependencies of reproductive biology make entirely predictable from a nutritional standpoint — the triage hierarchy deprioritizing reproductive function when the system is operating below the threshold of sufficiency. Early metabolic syndrome — insulin resistance, visceral adiposity, and dyslipidemia in people who are not yet thirty — is the energy and methylation story of this book playing out in a younger body that was never given the raw materials to regulate glucose and lipid metabolism correctly.

This is not a generation that is making worse lifestyle choices than their parents. It is a generation that inherited a more depleted starting point, faces a higher physiological demand, and is being failed by the same diagnostic framework that failed Margaret — a framework that sees each of these presentations as a separate condition requiring a separate specialist and a separate intervention, rather than as convergent signals from a single orchestra playing poorly across multiple sections simultaneously.

Clinicians should take notice. When a twenty-six-year-old presents with gray temples, myopia that worsened rapidly through adolescence, anxiety unresponsive to SSRIs, ADHD managed with stimulants whose response has plateaued, fatigue that no standard panel explains, a gut that reacts to an expanding list of foods, skin that has never fully cleared, and cycles that have never been regular — this is not a collection of unrelated complaints. It is the triage hierarchy operating ahead of schedule in a body that started the race already in deficit. The questions this book asks of Margaret are not questions for the fifty-year-old alone. They belong in every clinical encounter, at every age, with every patient whose multi-system presentation has outpaced medicine's willingness to look upstream.

The orchestra is playing poorly earlier. The seats have been empty longer. And Margaret's children cannot afford to wait decades for medicine to notice.

V. The Weight That Will Not Move

No consequence of the Invisible Famine is more visible, or more misunderstood, than the one written on the scale. Enormous effort and expense go into the project of losing weight — diet plan after plan, each promising the discipline the last one lacked — and most of it fails. The failure is almost always read the same way: as a shortage of willpower. The hypothesis of this book reads it differently. A body running the famine response is not storing fat *despite* the diet; it is storing fat because of the environment the diet is imposed on — nutrient-poor food that the nutrient sensors register as scarcity. Restricting calories on that same food does not resolve the signal. It deepens it. Told once again that lean months have arrived, the body defends its stores more tenaciously, slows its expenditure, and sharpens its hunger. The dieter is not fighting their weakness. They are fighting two million years of evolutionary logic, with a strategy that confirms the body's fear rather than relieving it.

This is why the weight so often will not move, and why, when it does, it so often returns. The instrument that governs it — the leptin signal that should say *enough* — has been desensitized by the very depletion the diet leaves untouched. Willpower cannot reach a broken satiety circuit, and calorie counting cannot restore a nutrient the food never contained. It is not that eating less never matters; it is that eating less of the wrong thing asks the body to surrender its reserves in the middle of what it believes is a famine — and the body was built to refuse. The question the hypothesis poses is not how to eat less, but how to end the famine: to give the nutrient sensors the abundance they have been signaling for, so the response they are running can finally stand down. Weight, in this framing, is not the problem to be solved. It is a symptom of a problem the scale was never able to name.

VI. What Medicine Would Look Like If It Asked the Right Questions

The medicine described in this book does not replace the medicine that currently exists. It augments it — adding an upstream layer of investigation that the current system has been structurally unable to provide.

In this augmented medicine, a patient presenting with Margaret's constellation of symptoms — multi-system complaints spanning cardiovascular, endocrine, neurological, gastrointestinal, and dermatological systems — would trigger a different set of questions. Not: which specialist should see each complaint? But: what single upstream story might explain all of them simultaneously? And what nutritional assessment would be required to tell that story?

The assessment would include: RBC magnesium, not serum magnesium. Serum and RBC copper alongside zinc, not copper or zinc alone. RBC selenium alongside glutathione. 25(OH)D alongside PTH and magnesium. Free T3 and free T4 alongside TSH, with selenium status in the interpretation. Anti-TPO antibody titres in the context of selenium and vitamin D. Fasting homocysteine alongside folate, B12, B6, and riboflavin. RBC fatty acid profile with omega-3 index. Plasma amino acids including glycine, taurine, and cysteine. Stool microbiome assessment alongside lactulose-mannitol ratio for gut permeability. Undercarboxylated osteocalcin for K2 status. A comprehensive dietary history focused specifically on amino acid sources, fat composition, fiber diversity, and fermented food intake.

This assessment would not fit in a seven-minute appointment. It would not be reimbursed by current billing structures. It would require a physician trained to interpret it and a clinical framework within which to act on the findings. None of these conditions currently exist in the standard clinical encounter. All of them are achievable with changes in training, incentives, and clinical culture that the evidence now clearly justifies.

VII. The Pioneers Revisited

The scientists honored in the Giants chapter each found a piece of this picture. Lonsdale at the Krebs cycle gate. Pauling in the oxidative stress of the arterial wall. Hoffer in the NAD+ chemistry of the psychiatric ward. Price in the fat-soluble vitamin content of the traditional diet. Klevay in the copper dependency of the cardiac muscle. Ames in the triage logic that explains how subclinical insufficiency produces long-term harm without announcing itself. Williams in the biochemical individuality that means no two people have identical nutritional requirements.

Each of them was pointing at part of an orchestra they could not fully see. The instruments they identified were real. The sections they missed were not fictitious — they simply fell outside the narrow beam of a scientific career necessarily focused on depth rather than breadth. The complete picture required someone to stand at a sufficient distance from each individual instrument to hear the full concert: to hear Lonsdale's thiamine at the Krebs cycle gate and simultaneously hear the copper at the terminal gate of the electron transport chain; to hear Pauling's vitamin C in the arterial wall and simultaneously hear the K2 and magnesium whose absence allows calcium to harden that wall; to hear Hoffer's niacin in the psychiatric ward and simultaneously hear the omega-3 in the neuronal membrane and the methylfolate at the B6-dependent serotonin synthesis step.

The complete picture is what this book has attempted to provide. Not a refutation of the pioneers — a completion of their work. The orchestra they described was real. It was simply larger, more interconnected, and more dependent on the whole than any of their individual discoveries fully conveyed.

VIII. The Orchestra Playing Well

What does optimal nutritional status actually feel like? It is worth naming, because the book has spent fourteen chapters describing what happens when the orchestra is impaired. What does a well-tuned orchestra produce?

Energy that is consistent and renewable — not the caffeine-dependent peak-and-crash pattern of the energy-deficient, but a baseline vitality that persists through demands and recovers after them. Sleep that comes readily and is restorative — the magnesium-adequate, GABA-sufficient, melatonin-synthesizing sleep of a nervous system that has what it needs. Mood that is stable and resilient — not the absence of emotion, but the neurochemical infrastructure to process experience without being destabilized by it. Cognitive function that is sharp and sustained — the DHA-rich, B12-replete, methylation-adequate brain of someone whose mental raw materials are present. Immune function that defends without overreacting — the vitamin D-modulated, zinc-adequate, omega-3-balanced immune system that kills pathogens, tolerates self, and resolves inflammation when its work is done. Structural integrity that holds — the copper-cross-linked, vitamin C-completed, K2-directed calcium architecture of a body that heals efficiently and ages with dignity.

These are not aspirational states reserved for the supremely healthy or the nutritionally obsessed. They are the biological default of a body that is given what it needs — the baseline that the species evolved on and that was available to most humans throughout most of human history. They are the state that the modern food environment, the low-fat dietary era, the antibiotic era, the chronic stress of contemporary life, and the processed food industry have conspired to make unusual rather than normal. They are recoverable. That is the message of this book.

IX. What Margaret Deserved

Margaret deserved a clinician who, when she described her fatigue, her anxiety, her bleeding gums, her thyroid medication that controlled her TSH but not her symptoms, her five medications, and her years of accumulating diagnoses without explanations — heard not five separate problems requiring five separate prescriptions, but one story requiring one investigation.

She deserved a conversation about her diet — specifically about the nutrients it was and was not providing, about the gut that was or was not absorbing them, about the medications that were or were not depleting them. She deserved blood tests that measured what her cells were actually doing rather than what her blood's reference range suggested. She deserved an explanation of why the orchestra was playing so poorly — not five separate explanations for five separate instruments, but one explanation for one orchestra.

She deserved to know that her bleeding gums were not a failure of dental hygiene but a signal from her collagen architecture. That her fatigue was not laziness or stress but her energy machinery running without adequate fuel. That her anxiety was not a psychiatric condition requiring indefinite medication but a nervous system impaired by B-vitamin depletion, omega-3 insufficiency, and a gut-brain axis disrupted by a microbiome that four antibiotic courses had damaged and no subsequent intervention had rebuilt. That her thyroid medication was replacing the hormone without addressing the selenium that would reduce the antibodies destroying her gland. That her hypertension might respond to magnesium in ways that her current medications, which deplete magnesium, could never reach.

She deserved the questions this book asks. Not the answers — every person's answers are individual, biochemically specific, and require clinical assessment. But the questions. The upstream questions. The questions that see the orchestra behind the noise.

> *The body has not changed. The orchestra was always there — all sixty musicians, all fourteen sections, all the dependencies and interactions and triage hierarchies that this book has described. What has changed is the world around the orchestra: the food that depletes it, the medications that impair it, the medical system that hears only its loudest failures and treats them in isolation. Margaret is not a medical mystery. She is a musical one. And she deserved to be heard.*

X. The Questions Worth Asking — For Every Patient, for Every Reader

This book ends not with a protocol but with a set of questions. They are the questions that a nutritionally informed clinician would ask at the start of any investigation of multi-system chronic illness.

They are also the questions that any reader who recognizes themselves in Margaret's story might begin to pursue.

Energy: Has anyone measured RBC magnesium, not serum magnesium? Has anyone assessed thiamine status functionally? Has anyone measured CoQ10, particularly if a beta-blocker or statin is being taken? Has anyone assessed copper alongside zinc rather than in isolation?

Gut: Is there a history of repeated antibiotic use without subsequent gut restoration? Is acid suppression medication being used long-term? Has gut permeability been assessed? Has microbiome diversity been measured?

Hormones: Has free T3 been measured alongside TSH in thyroid management? Has selenium status been assessed in the context of Hashimoto's antibodies? Has magnesium status been assessed in the context of insulin resistance?

Neurology and mood: Has homocysteine been measured? Has methylfolate status been assessed? Has the omega-3 index been measured? Has B12 functional status been confirmed with methylmalonic acid?

Immunity: Has vitamin D been measured and systematically corrected to an adequate level? Has zinc been measured in the context of immune or autoimmune conditions? Has the inflammatory eicosanoid balance been considered in the context of the dietary omega-6:omega-3 ratio?

Structure: Has copper status been assessed in the context of osteoporosis or arterial disease? Has undercarboxylated osteocalcin been measured for vitamin K2 status? Has vitamin C been assessed in the context of cardiovascular risk or slow wound healing?

Protective compounds: Does the diet include cruciferous vegetables at least three times per week? Has macular pigment optical density been measured in anyone over fifty, particularly with a family history of macular degeneration? Has dietary spermidine intake been considered in the context of cardiovascular risk or cognitive aging? Has inositol been assessed as a therapeutic option in PCOS or insulin resistance? Has time spent outdoors been asked about — specifically morning light exposure — in anyone presenting with fatigue, mood disorder, or metabolic syndrome? Has the absence of phytonutrients from the diet been named as a problem in its own right, rather than left as the invisible background against which the named deficiencies are diagnosed?

These questions have answers. The answers require tests that exist. The tests require a clinician who has been asked to order them and a framework within which to interpret the results. That framework is this book.

What Margaret Truly Deserved

The Story That Could Have Been Different

Margaret's story did not have to end the way it ended.

Not with five medications and five diagnoses and three to five thousand dollars per year and a quiet, persistent sense that she was being managed rather than helped. Not with the fatigue that never lifted, the gums that kept bleeding, the skin that kept flaring, the anxiety that the medication contained but never resolved, the thyroid that the test said was fine while every cell in her body knew it was not.

The medicine that could have helped Margaret exists. It is not alternative medicine or fringe medicine or unproven medicine. It is nutritional biochemistry — as rigorous, as evidence-grounded, and as mechanistically precise as the pharmacology that her physicians applied to her downstream symptoms. The difference is that it asks different questions. Upstream questions. Questions about the orchestra behind the noise.

In the version of Margaret's story that this book imagines — the version she deserved — someone heard the orchestra rather than the individual instruments. Someone understood that her energy architects (Cluster 1) were working without adequate magnesium, copper, and CoQ10, and that three of her medications were deepening those depletions. Someone recognized that her gut gateway (Cluster 2) had been damaged by four antibiotic courses and three years of acid suppression, and that a compromised gateway was limiting the bioavailability of every other intervention. Someone looked at her microbiome (Cluster 3) and saw not a normal scope result but an ecosystem that had been repeatedly devastated and never restored, producing less butyrate, less serotonin precursor, and more systemic LPS endotoxemia than a healthy gut would allow. Someone measured her selenium and found it insufficient for the deiodinase enzymes of Cluster 6 converting her T4 to active T3 — and recognized simultaneously that the same selenium deficiency was allowing anti-TPO antibodies to continue destroying her gland. Someone assessed her homocysteine, checked her MTHFR status, and optimized the methylation network of Cluster 9 whose impairment was simultaneously elevating her cardiovascular risk and reducing the glutathione that protects every other system. Someone connected her bleeding gums to the structural architects of Cluster 5 — ascorbate, copper, and glycine simultaneously — rather than to her flossing technique. And someone measured her omega-3 index and found it at four percent, recognizing that the neuronal and immune membranes of Clusters 7 and 13 were operating in a chronically pro-inflammatory fatty acid environment that no pharmaceutical could reach. And someone noticed that her diet had quietly eliminated an entire class of protective biological inputs — the sulforaphane-inducible enzymes that were leaving her phase II detoxification running below capacity, the lutein and zeaxanthin that her macular pigment was quietly depleting, the spermidine that her cellular maintenance machinery had stopped receiving —

and addressed them not with a pharmaceutical substitute but with the foods that had always supplied them.

What Margaret lived through has a name. She was never starving — the shelves were full, the plates were loaded — and that was precisely the problem. She was living through the Invisible Famine: abundance without nourishment, a body reading plenty as scarcity and quietly powering itself down. The tragedy was not that the famine was severe. It was that it was invisible — to her, to her physicians, to a system never trained to look for it. The medicine she deserved did only one thing differently: it made the famine visible. And a hunger, once seen, can be fed.

In this imagined version, Margaret's fatigue lifts over months — not all at once, not dramatically, but progressively, as the energy machinery receives what it was missing. Her anxiety reduces as magnesium-dependent NMDA receptor regulation improves and as the gut-brain axis rebuilds on a restored microbiome and adequate methylfolate. Her gums stop bleeding as her collagen architecture is supported with adequate ascorbate, copper, and glycine. Her thyroid symptoms diminish as the selenium that reduces her anti-TPO antibodies and enables T4-to-T3 conversion is replenished. Her skin condition — which responded to emollient creams but never resolved — quiets as her vitamin A status improves the mucosal and epidermal differentiation that was contributing to it.

She is still on some of her medications. The restoration of nutritional sufficiency does not instantly reverse years of structural and metabolic change. But the medications do more because the system they are acting on is better supported.

Margaret, in this version, does not exit the medical system. She becomes a different kind of patient within it — one who brings upstream information to downstream conversations, who asks the questions this book has given her, who understands that her conditions are not a collection of separate failures but a single orchestral story that can be heard, interpreted, and addressed.

This is what medicine could be. What it should be. What the evidence — decades of it, across hundreds of laboratories and clinical settings, by the pioneers honored in this book and by the researchers who have built on their work — already supports.

The orchestra was always there. Every musician was always essential. The concert was always possible.

Margaret deserved to hear it.

—

Acknowledgements

This book was shaped by two decades of reading, observing, and listening — to the scientific literature, to family members, to friends, to colleagues, and to the countless people who have described, with remarkable consistency, the same experience: years of appointments, folders of normal test results, and one question medicine never answered. Not what do I have — but what is causing it. They were not imagining their symptoms. They were navigating a system not designed to look for where the answers were. This book is an attempt to point toward them.

The Scientists Who Looked Upstream

Every insight in this book rests on researchers, who argued, against institutional resistance, that nutritional insufficiency sat at the root of diseases medicine was treating as primary conditions. Each found a critical piece of the puzzle. This book is indebted to all of them.

Dr. Derrick Lonsdale — whose five decades of work on thiamine and the ATP gateway is foundational to this book's central argument. He was largely ignored by mainstream medicine. He was right.

Linus Pauling — who understood before almost anyone that the RDA represented a floor for avoiding deficiency, not a ceiling for optimal function, and that chronic disease lived in the gap between them.

Dr. Abram Hoffer — who demonstrated that NAD+ depletion drove psychiatric disease that medicine had labeled without ever investigating its nutritional root.

Dr. Weston A. Price — who documented, with photographic precision, the physical degeneration that followed dietary industrialization across populations worldwide.

Dr. Leslie Klevay — who built the cardiovascular case for copper with careful, decades-long research that deserved far more attention than it received.

Dr. Bruce Ames — whose triage theory — that subclinical micronutrient insufficiency forces the body to prioritize survival over long-term maintenance — is among the most elegant frameworks in nutritional medicine.

Roger J. Williams — whose concept of biochemical individuality established that human nutritional requirements vary dramatically between individuals, and that the gap between the population average and any given person's true requirement is where chronic disease quietly develops. His insight that nutrients function as a team — interdependent, mutually regulating — is the intellectual foundation of this book's cluster architecture.

Joseph Goldberger — who proved, against fierce institutional resistance, that pellagra was a disease of dietary deficiency rather than infection, and whose willingness to challenge the medical consensus of his day is the tradition this book attempts to honor.

Dr. Emanuel Cheraskin — whose concept of the optimum nutrient intake — not merely the absence of deficiency disease but the intake associated with peak physiological function — gave clinical language to what this book argues across fourteen clusters.

Dr. Andrew Saul — who spent 35 years making orthomolecular medicine accessible to patients and practitioners alike, founding the Orthomolecular Medicine News Service and building the bridge between the science these pioneers produced and the people who needed it most. His website DoctorYourself.com — a vast, freely accessible archive of nutritional science and age-old clinical literature — was an invaluable resource during the research for this book. His documentary Food Matters was an early inspiration.

Christiaan Eijkman — whose 1897 discovery that beriberi was a disease of diet, not infection, established the principle this book has tried to honor at every turn: that a condition assumed to be one thing is often, on closer inspection, something else entirely.

Denis Burkitt — whose comparison of disease rates across continents revealed what no single-patient study could have shown, and whose method of looking at populations rather than individuals runs through every chapter of this book.

George and Mildred Burr — who together identified the omega-3 and omega-6 essential fatty acids, though only one of their names is widely remembered. This book tries, in its own small way, to correct that.

A Note on Claude

This book was researched and written in collaboration with Claude, an artificial intelligence developed by Anthropic. Claude contributed cross-domain synthesis — connecting biochemistry, clinical medicine, nutritional science, and medical history simultaneously — at a scale and speed that traditional research methods cannot match.

Personal Gratitude

To the researchers and clinicians who have pursued root-cause medicine at the margins of a system not designed to reward it — this book attempts to bring your work to the audience it deserves.

To everyone who has been sick, spent, and praying for answers — the answers were there all along. They just required someone to look upstream.

"The important thing is not to stop questioning."
— Albert Einstein

A Note on Sources

This book is a work of medical non-fiction. It is not a systematic review, a meta-analysis, or a clinical guideline. It is a synthesis of evidence drawn from peer-reviewed biochemistry, physiology, and clinical nutrition literature, presented in a form accessible to the general reader without sacrificing scientific accuracy.

The references that follow are organized by cluster. They support the specific quantitative claims, named studies, and clinical evidence cited in the text and in the For the Clinically Curious sections. They are not exhaustive — the science underlying each cluster spans decades of primary literature, and a complete bibliography would double the length of the book. The citations here represent the primary sources for the book's most specific claims: the named trials, the percentage figures, the mechanistic papers, and the key reviews that anchor each cluster's argument.

Readers seeking a broader engagement with the literature are directed to the review articles cited, many of which contain comprehensive reference lists spanning the full depth of each topic. Where a claim rests on established biochemistry rather than a specific study — the role of thiamine pyrophosphate in the pyruvate dehydrogenase complex, the structure of the electron transport chain, the amino acid composition of collagen — standard biochemistry texts and authoritative reviews are the appropriate sources, and individual citations are not provided for widely accepted mechanistic facts.

All cited studies were accessed and verified. Where a study is described with specific numerical findings — percentage reductions, effect sizes, population frequencies — those figures reflect the published primary source.

References

Opening: The Map We Were Given

Preface: Why I Wrote This Book

On leptin as the primary adiposity and satiety signal:

Friedman JM. Leptin and the endocrine control of energy balance. Nature Metabolism. 2019;1(8):754-764.

On leptin resistance — mechanism and consequences for appetite regulation:

Myers MG, Leibel RL, Seeley RJ, Schwartz MW. Obesity and leptin resistance: distinguishing cause from effect. Trends in Endocrinology and Metabolism. 2010;21(11):643-651.

On hypothalamic nutrient sensing, famine signaling, and metabolic triage:

Lustig RH. Fructose: metabolic, hedonic, and societal parallels with ethanol. Journal of the American Dietetic Association. 2010;110(9):1307-1321.

On the Flexner Report and its consequences for nutritional medicine:

Flexner A. Medical Education in the United States and Canada: A Report to the Carnegie Foundation for the Advancement of Teaching. Carnegie Foundation; 1910.

Starr P. The Social Transformation of American Medicine. Basic Books; 1982.

Ornish D, Topol EJ. Lifestyle medicine is the standard of care for preventive cardiology. Lancet. 2024;403(10440):1989-1992.

On pharmaceutical funding of clinical research and publication bias:

Lexchin J, Bero LA, Djulbegovic B, Clark O. Pharmaceutical industry sponsorship and research outcome and quality: systematic review. BMJ. 2003;326(7400):1167-1170.

Bekelman JE, Li Y, Gross CP. Scope and impact of financial conflicts of interest in biomedical research: a systematic review. JAMA. 2003;289(4):454-465.

On RCT methodological limitations in nutritional research:

Mozaffarian D. Dietary and policy priorities for cardiovascular disease, diabetes, and obesity: a comprehensive review. Circulation. 2016;133(2):187-225.

Ioannidis JP. Implausible results in human nutrition research. BMJ. 2013;347:f6698.

Standing on the Shoulders of Giants

On Derrick Lonsdale and thiamine deficiency:

Lonsdale D. A review of the biochemistry, metabolism and clinical benefits of thiamin(e) and its derivatives. Evidence-Based Complementary and Alternative Medicine. 2006;3(1):49-59.

Lonsdale D, Marrs C. Thiamine Deficiency Disease, Dysautonomia, and High Calorie Malnutrition. Academic Press; 2017.

On Linus Pauling and orthomolecular medicine:

Pauling L. Orthomolecular psychiatry. Science. 1968;160(3825):265-271.

Pauling L. How to Live Longer and Feel Better. W.H. Freeman; 1986.

On Abram Hoffer and niacin:

Hoffer A, Osmond H. The Chemical Basis of Clinical Psychiatry. Charles C Thomas; 1960.

Hoffer A. Niacin Therapy in Psychiatry. Charles C Thomas; 1962.

On Weston A. Price and fat-soluble vitamins:

Price WA. Nutrition and Physical Degeneration. Paul B. Hoeber; 1939.

On Leslie Klevay and copper:

Klevay LM. Cardiovascular disease from copper deficiency — a history. Journal of Nutrition. 2000;130(2S Suppl):489S-492S.

Klevay LM. IHD from copper deficiency. Acta Pharmacologica Sinica. 2004;25(12):1512-1520.

On Bruce Ames and the triage theory:

Ames BN. Low micronutrient intake may accelerate the degenerative diseases of aging through allocation of scarce micronutrients by triage. Proceedings of the National Academy of Sciences. 2006;103(47):17589-17594.

McCann JC, Ames BN. Vitamin K, an example of triage theory: is micronutrient inadequacy linked to diseases of aging? American Journal of Clinical Nutrition. 2009;90(4):889-907.

On Roger Williams and biochemical individuality:

Williams RJ. Biochemical Individuality: The Basis for the Genetotrophic Concept. Wiley; 1956.

On Otto Warburg and cellular respiration and cancer metabolism:

Warburg O. On the origin of cancer cells. Science. 1956;123(3191):309-314.

On Emanuel Cheraskin and predictive, orthomolecular medicine:

Cheraskin E, Ringsdorf WM. Predictive Medicine: A Study in Strategy. Pacific Press Publishing Association; 1973.

On Christiaan Eijkman and the discovery of the antineuritic factor:

Eijkman C. Antineuritic vitamin and beriberi. Nobel Lecture, 1929. In: Nobel Lectures, Physiology or Medicine 1922-1941. Elsevier; 1965.

On Denis Burkitt, dietary fiber, and colorectal cancer:

Burkitt DP. Epidemiology of cancer of the colon and rectum. Cancer. 1971;28(1):3-13.

On George and Mildred Burr and the discovery of essential fatty acids:

Burr GO, Burr MM. A new deficiency disease produced by the rigid exclusion of fat from the diet. Journal of Biological Chemistry. 1929;82:345-367.

Burr GO, Burr MM. On the nature and role of the fatty acids essential in nutrition. Journal of Biological Chemistry. 1930;86:587-621.

On Andrew Saul and orthomolecular medicine outreach:

Saul AW. Doctor Yourself: Natural Healing That Works. Basic Health Publications; 2003.

Cluster 1: The Energy Architects

On thiamine, the pyruvate dehydrogenase complex, and subclinical deficiency:

Lonsdale D. Thiamine and magnesium deficiencies: keys to disease. Medical Hypotheses. 2015;84(2):129-134.

Maslewska G, Lonsdale D. Metabolic effects of high calorie malnutrition and their relevance to thiamine deficiency. Nutrients. 2021;13(9):3067.

Hirsch M, Hannoun C, Hort J. Thiamine deficiency in developed countries — still a problem. European Journal of Neurology. 2006;13(10):1052-1058.

On riboflavin and the electron transport chain:

Powers HJ. Riboflavin (vitamin B2) and health. American Journal of Clinical Nutrition. 2003;77(6):1352-1360.

On niacin, NAD+ depletion and pellagra:

Gasperi V, Sibilano M, Savini I, Catani MV. Niacin in the central nervous system: an update of biological aspects and clinical applications. International Journal of Molecular Sciences. 2019;20(4):974.

Abdelmalek MF. Nonalcoholic fatty liver disease and niacin: from pathogenesis to treatment. Current Opinion in Gastroenterology. 2017;33(3):154-161.

On magnesium — RBC vs. serum measurement, and MgATP:

Workinger JL, Doyle RP, Bortz J. Challenges in the diagnosis of magnesium status. Nutrients. 2018;10(9):1202.

de Baaij JH, Hoenderop JG, Bindels RJ. Magnesium in man: implications for health and disease. Physiological Reviews. 2015;95(1):1-46.

Altura BM, Altura BT. Magnesium and cardiovascular biology: an important link between cardiovascular risk factors and atherogenesis. Cellular and Molecular Biology Research. 1995;41(5):347-359.

On iron-sulfur clusters and ETC function independent of anemia:

Rouault TA. The role of iron regulatory proteins in mammalian iron homeostasis and disease. Nature Chemical Biology. 2006;2(8):406-414.

Zimmermann MB, Hurrell RF. Nutritional iron deficiency. Lancet. 2007;370(9586):511-520.

On copper at Complex IV (cytochrome c oxidase):

Tsukihara T, Aoyama H, Yamashita E, et al. The whole structure of the 13-subunit oxidized cytochrome c oxidase at 2.8 Å. Science. 1996;272(5265):1136-1144.

Leary SC, Winge DR, Cobine PA. 'Pulling the plug' on cellular copper: the role of mitochondria in copper export. Biochimica et Biophysica Acta. 2009;1793(1):146-153.

On CoQ10 depletion by statins:

Littarru GP, Tiano L. Bioenergetic and antioxidant properties of coenzyme Q10: recent developments. Molecular Biotechnology. 2007;37(1):31-37.

Päivä H, Thelen KM, Van Coster R, et al. High-dose statins and skeletal muscle metabolism in humans: a randomized, controlled trial. Clinical Pharmacology & Therapeutics. 2005;78(1):60-68.

On PQQ and mitochondrial biogenesis:

Rucker R, Chowanadisai W, Nakano M. Potential physiological importance of pyrroloquinoline quinone. Alternative Medicine Review. 2009;14(3):268-277.

Harris CB, Chowanadisai W, Mishchuk DO, et al. Dietary pyrroloquinoline quinone (PQQ) alters indicators of inflammation and mitochondrial-related metabolism in human subjects. Journal of Nutritional Biochemistry. 2013;24(12):2076-2084.

Cluster 2: The Master Gateway

On tight junction proteins, zonulin, and intestinal permeability measurement:

Fasano A. Zonulin and its regulation of intestinal barrier function: the biological door to inflammation, autoimmunity, and cancer. Physiological Reviews. 2011;91(1):151-175.

Fasano A. Intestinal permeability and its regulation by zonulin: diagnostic and therapeutic implications. Clinical Gastroenterology and Hepatology. 2012;10(10):1096-1100.

Turner JR. Intestinal mucosal barrier function in health and disease. Nature Reviews Immunology. 2009;9(11):799-809.

On LPS endotoxemia and metabolic disease:

Cani PD, Amar J, Iglesias MA, et al. Metabolic endotoxemia initiates obesity and insulin resistance. Diabetes. 2007;56(7):1761-1772.

Laugerette F, Furet JP, Debard C, et al. Oil composition of high-fat diet affects metabolic inflammation differently in connection with endotoxin receptors in mice. American Journal of Physiology — Endocrinology and Metabolism. 2012;302(3):E374-E386.

On phosphatidylcholine supplementation in ulcerative colitis:

Stremmel W, Merle U, Zahn A, et al. Retarded release phosphatidylcholine benefits patients with chronic active ulcerative colitis. Gut. 2005;54(7):966-971.

Stremmel W, Braun A, Hanemann A, et al. Delayed release phosphatidylcholine in chronic-active ulcerative colitis: a randomized, double-blinded, dose finding study. Journal of Clinical Gastroenterology. 2010;44(5):e101-e107.

On vitamin D and gut barrier function:

Kong J, Zhang Z, Musch MW, et al. Novel role of the vitamin D receptor in maintaining the integrity of the intestinal mucosal barrier. American Journal of Physiology — Gastrointestinal and Liver Physiology. 2008;294(1):G208-G216.

On zinc and tight junction integrity:

Finamore A, Massimi M, Conti Devirgiliis L, Mengheri E. Zinc deficiency induces membrane barrier damage and increases neutrophil transmigration in Caco-2 cells. Journal of Nutrition. 2008;138(9):1664-1670.

On butyrate, HDAC inhibition, and colonic health:

Donohoe DR, Collins LB, Wali A, et al. The Warburg effect dictates the mechanism of butyrate-mediated histone acetylation and cell proliferation. Molecular Cell. 2012;48(4):612-626.

Canani RB, Costanzo MD, Leone L, et al. Potential beneficial effects of butyrate in intestinal and extraintestinal diseases. World Journal of Gastroenterology. 2011;17(12):1519-1528.

Cluster 3: The Garden Within

On antibiotic effects on the microbiome:

Dethlefsen L, Huse S, Sogin ML, Relman DA. The pervasive effects of an antibiotic on the human gut microbiota, as revealed by deep 16S rRNA sequencing. PLoS Biology. 2008;6(11):e280.

Jernberg C, Löfmark S, Edlund C, Jansson JK. Long-term impacts of antibiotic exposure on the human intestinal microbiota. Microbiology. 2010;156(11):3216-3223.

On the Stanford fermented food RCT:

Wastyk HC, Fragiadakis GK, Perelman D, et al. Gut-microbiota-targeted diets modulate human immune status. Cell. 2021;184(16):4137-4153.e14.

On microbiome and psychiatric conditions:

Cryan JF, O'Riordan KJ, Cowan CS, et al. The microbiota-gut-brain axis. Physiological Reviews. 2019;99(4):1877-2013.

Simpson CA, Diaz-Arteche C, Eliby D, et al. The gut microbiota in anxiety and depression — a systematic review. Clinical Psychology Review. 2021;83:101943.

On the tryptophan-kynurenine pathway and IDO activation in depression:

Dantzer R, O'Connor JC, Freund GG, Johnson RW, Kelley KW. From inflammation to sickness and depression: when the immune system subjugates the brain. Nature Reviews Neuroscience. 2008;9(1):46-56.

Myint AM, Kim YK. Network beyond IDO in psychiatric disorders: revisited. Frontiers in Neuroscience. 2014;8:110.

On Akkermansia muciniphila and metabolic health:

Plovier H, Everard A, Druart C, et al. A purified membrane protein from Akkermansia muciniphila or the pasteurised bacterium improves metabolism in obese and diabetic mice. Nature Medicine. 2017;23(1):107-113.

Depommier C, Everard A, Druart C, et al. Supplementation with Akkermansia muciniphila in overweight and obese human volunteers: a proof-of-concept exploratory study. Nature Medicine. 2019;25(7):1096-1103.

On urolithin A and mitophagy:

Andreux PA, Blanco-Bose W, Ryu D, et al. The mitophagy activator urolithin A is safe and induces a molecular signature of improved mitochondrial and cellular health in humans. Nature Metabolism. 2019;1(6):595-603.

On diversity of plant foods and microbiome diversity:

McDonald D, Hyde E, Debelius JW, et al. American Gut: an open platform for citizen science microbiome research. mSystems. 2018;3(3):e00031-18.

Cluster 4: The Antioxidant Shield

On the glutathione regeneration cascade and G6PD deficiency:

Lushchak VI. Glutathione homeostasis and functions: potential targets for medical interventions. Journal of Amino Acids. 2012;2012:736837.

Cappellini MD, Fiorelli G. Glucose-6-phosphate dehydrogenase deficiency. Lancet. 2008;371(9606):64-74.

On the SOD2 Val16Ala variant (rs4880) and manganese:

Sutton A, Khoury H, Prip-Buus C, et al. The Ala16Val genetic dimorphism modulates the import of human manganese superoxide dismutase into rat liver mitochondria. Pharmacogenetics. 2003;13(3):145-157.

Ambrosone CB, Freudenheim JL, Thompson PA, et al. Manganese superoxide dismutase (MnSOD) genetic polymorphisms, dietary antioxidants, and risk of breast cancer. Cancer Research. 1999;59(3):602-606.

On 8-OHdG as a biomarker of oxidative DNA damage:

Valavanidis A, Vlachogianni T, Fiotakis C. 8-hydroxy-2'-deoxyguanosine (8-OHdG): a critical biomarker of oxidative stress and carcinogenesis. Journal of Environmental Science and Health. 2009;27(2):120-139.

On NAC and glycine as glutathione precursors — the Kumar trial:

Kumar P, Liu C, Suliburk J, et al. Supplementing glycine and N-acetylcysteine (GlyNAC) in older adults improves glutathione deficiency, oxidative stress, mitochondrial dysfunction, inflammation, insulin resistance, endothelial dysfunction, genotoxicity, muscle strength, and cognition: results of a pilot clinical trial. Journal of Gerontology. 2023;78(1):75-89.

On selenium and thyroid function (deiodinase):

Schomburg L. Selenium, selenoproteins and the thyroid gland: interactions in health and disease. Nature Reviews Endocrinology. 2012;8(3):160-171.

On the antioxidant network and LDL oxidation in cardiovascular disease:

Stocker R, Keaney JF Jr. Role of oxidative modifications in atherosclerosis. Physiological Reviews. 2004;84(4):1381-1478.

Cluster 5: The Structural Architects

On lysyl oxidase, copper, and collagen cross-linking:

Lucero HA, Kagan HM. Lysyl oxidase: an oxidative enzyme and effector of cell function. Cellular and Molecular Life Sciences. 2006;63(19-20):2304-2316.

Rucker RB, Kosonen T, Clegg MS, et al. Copper, lysyl oxidase, and extracellular matrix protein cross-linking. American Journal of Clinical Nutrition. 1998;67(5 Suppl):996S-1002S.

On Menkes disease and occipital horn syndrome as copper deficiency models:

Tümer Z. An overview and update of ATP7A mutations leading to Menkes disease and occipital horn syndrome. Human Mutation. 2013;34(3):417-429.

On bisphosphonates, bone matrix quality, and atypical femoral fractures:

Odvina CV, Zerwekh JE, Rao DS, et al. Severely suppressed bone turnover: a potential complication of alendronate therapy. Journal of Clinical Endocrinology & Metabolism. 2005;90(3):1294-1301.

Shane E, Burr D, Ebeling PR, et al. Atypical subtrochanteric and diaphyseal femoral fractures: report of a task force of the American Society for Bone and Mineral Research. Journal of Bone and Mineral Research. 2010;25(11):2267-2294.

On vitamin K2 (menaquinone), osteocalcin, and cardiovascular outcomes — the Rotterdam Study:

Geleijnse JM, Vermeer C, Grobbee DE, et al. Dietary intake of menaquinone is associated with a reduced risk of coronary heart disease: the Rotterdam Study. Journal of Nutrition. 2004;134(11):3100-3105.

Vermeer C. Vitamin K: the effect on health beyond coagulation — an overview. Food & Nutrition Research. 2012;56:5329.

On matrix Gla protein (MGP) and arterial calcification:

Schurgers LJ, Teunissen KJ, Hamulyák K, et al. Vitamin K-containing dietary supplements: comparison of synthetic vitamin K1 and natto-derived menaquinone-7. Blood. 2007;109(8):3279-3283.

Cranenburg EC, Schurgers LJ, Vermeer C. Vitamin K: the coagulation vitamin that became omnipotent. Thrombosis and Hemostasis. 2007;98(1):120-125.

On glycine requirements and deficiency in modern diets:

Meléndez-Hevia E, De Paz-Lugo P, Cornish-Bowden A, Cárdenas ML. A weak link in metabolism: the metabolic capacity for glycine biosynthesis does not satisfy the need for collagen synthesis. Journal of Biosciences. 2009;34(6):853-872.

On silicon and bone mineralisation:

Jugdaohsingh R. Silicon and bone health. Journal of Nutrition, Health & Aging. 2007;11(2):99-110. Jugdaohsingh R, Anderson SH, Tucker KL, et al. Dietary silicon intake and absorption. American Journal of Clinical Nutrition. 2002;75(5):887-893.

Cluster 6: The Hormonal Regulators

On selenium, deiodinase enzymes, and thyroid hormone conversion:

Köhrle J. Selenium and the thyroid. Current Opinion in Endocrinology, Diabetes and Obesity. 2015;22(5):392-401.

Schomburg L, Köhrle J. On the importance of selenium and iodine metabolism for thyroid hormone biosynthesis and human health. Molecular Nutrition & Food Research. 2008;52(11):1235-1246.

On selenium supplementation and anti-TPO antibody reduction in Hashimoto's — the systematic review and meta-analysis:

Wichman J, Winther KH, Bonnema SJ, Hegedüs L. Selenium supplementation significantly reduces thyroid autoantibody levels in patients with chronic autoimmune thyroiditis: a systematic review and meta-analysis. Thyroid. 2016;26(12):1681-1692.

van Zuuren EJ, Albusta AY, Fedorowicz Z, Carter B, Pijl H. Selenium supplementation for Hashimoto's thyroiditis: summary of a Cochrane systematic review. European Thyroid Journal. 2014;3(1):25-31.

On chromodulin and insulin signaling:

Vincent JB. The biochemistry of chromium. Journal of Nutrition. 2000;130(4):715-718.

Cefalu WT, Hu FB. Role of chromium in human health and in diabetes. Diabetes Care. 2004;27(11):2741-2751.

On magnesium and insulin resistance — the bidirectional relationship:

Guerrero-Romero F, Rodríguez-Morán M. Magnesium improves the beta-cell function to compensate variation of insulin sensitivity: double-blind, randomized clinical trial. European Journal of Clinical Investigation. 2011;41(4):405-410.

Barbagallo M, Dominguez LJ. Magnesium and type 2 diabetes. World Journal of Diabetes. 2015;6(10):1152-1157.

On the INTERSALT study and potassium and blood pressure:

Intersalt Cooperative Research Group. Intersalt: an international study of electrolyte excretion and blood pressure. Results for 24 hour urinary sodium and potassium excretion. BMJ. 1988;297(6644):319-328.

On thyroid peroxidase and iron dependency:

Zimmermann MB, Köhrle J. The impact of iron and selenium deficiencies on iodine and thyroid metabolism: biochemistry and relevance to public health. Thyroid. 2002;12(10):867-878.

Cluster 7: The Neurological Foundations

On MTHFR C677T, BH4, and neurotransmitter synthesis:

Stahl SM. L-methylfolate: a vitamin for your monoamines. Journal of Clinical Psychiatry. 2008;69(9):1352-1353.

Papakostas GI, Shelton RC, Zajecka JM, et al. L-methylfolate as adjunctive therapy for SSRI-resistant major depression: results of two randomized, double-blind, parallel-sequential trials. American Journal of Psychiatry. 2012;169(12):1267-1274.

On lithium at trace dietary levels — the meta-analysis:

Memon A, Rogers I, Fitzsimmons SM, et al. Association between naturally occurring lithium in drinking water and suicide mortality: systematic review and meta-analysis. British Journal of Psychiatry. 2020;217(6):667-678.

On copper deficiency myelopathy and misdiagnosis:

Prodan CI, Holland NR, Wisdom PJ, et al. CNS demyelination associated with copper deficiency and hyperzincemia. Neurology. 2002;59(9):1453-1456.

Bhatt S, Bhatt BH, Vaidyanathan S, et al. Copper deficiency myelopathy in a patient taking zinc supplementation for hair loss. Practical Neurology. 2018;18(2):158-160.

On magnesium and the NMDA receptor — the clinical RCT:

Tarleton EK, Littenberg B, MacLean CD, Kennedy AG, Daley C. Role of magnesium supplementation in the treatment of depression: a randomized clinical trial. PLoS One. 2017;12(6):e0180067.

On DHA and neuronal membrane function:

Bazinet RP, Layé S. Polyunsaturated fatty acids and their metabolites in brain function and disease. Nature Reviews Neuroscience. 2014;15(12):771-785.

On B12 deficiency and subacute combined degeneration:

Stabler SP. Vitamin B12 deficiency. New England Journal of Medicine. 2013;368(2):149-160.

On serotonin synthesis and iron/B6 cofactors:

Youdim MB, Ben-Shachar D, Yehuda S. Putative biological mechanisms of the effect of iron deficiency on brain biochemistry and behavior. American Journal of Clinical Nutrition. 1989;50(3 Suppl):607-617.

Cluster 8: The Immune Architects

On vitamin D and Th17/Treg balance — molecular mechanism:

Mora JR, Iwata M, von Andrian UH. Vitamin effects on the immune system: vitamins A and D take center stage. Nature Reviews Immunology. 2008;8(9):685-698.

Prietl B, Treiber G, Pieber TR, Amrein K. Vitamin D and immune function. Nutrients. 2013;5(7):2502-2521.

On magnesium and LFA-1 T-cell cytotoxic function — the 2022 Cell paper:

Lötscher J, Martí i Líndez AA, Kirchhammer N, et al. Magnesium sensing via LFA-1 regulates CD8+ T cell cytotoxicity. Cell. 2022;185(4):585-602.e29.

On resolvins and protectins — the active resolution biology:

Serhan CN, Chiang N, Dalli J. The resolution code of acute inflammation: novel pro-resolving lipid mediators in resolution. Seminars in Immunology. 2015;27(3):200-215.

Serhan CN. Pro-resolving lipid mediators are leads for resolution physiology. Nature. 2014;510(7503):92-101.

On vitamin D latitude gradient and autoimmune disease:

Cantorna MT, Mahon BD. Mounting evidence for vitamin D as an environmental factor affecting autoimmune disease prevalence. Experimental Biology and Medicine. 2004;229(11):1136-1142.

On thymulin and zinc dependency:

Mocchegiani E, Muzzioli M, Giacconi R. Zinc, metallothioneins, immune responses, survival and aging. Biogerontology. 2000;1(2):133-143.

On omega-3 fatty acids and inflammatory resolution in autoimmune conditions:

Calder PC. Omega-3 fatty acids and inflammatory processes: from molecules to man. Biochemical Society Transactions. 2017;45(5):1105-1115.

Cluster 9: The Methylation Network

On MTHFR C677T enzyme biochemistry and population frequency:

Frosst P, Blom HJ, Milos R, et al. A candidate genetic risk factor for vascular disease: a common mutation in methylenetetrahydrofolate reductase. Nature Genetics. 1995;10(1):111-113.

Klerk M, Verhoef P, Clarke R, et al. MTHFR 677C→T polymorphism and risk of coronary heart disease: a meta-analysis. JAMA. 2002;288(16):2023-2031.

On riboflavin and MTHFR function — the clinical evidence:

McNulty H, Strain JJ, Pentieva K, Ward M. C1 metabolism and CVD outcomes in older adults. Proceedings of the Nutrition

Society. 2012;71(2):213-221.

On homocysteine and cardiovascular risk — the Homocysteine Studies Collaboration:

Homocysteine Studies Collaboration. Homocysteine and risk of ischemic heart disease and stroke: a meta-analysis. JAMA. 2002;288(16):2015-2022.

On SAMe in depression — the clinical evidence:

Papakostas GI, Mischoulon D, Shyu I, Alpert JE, Fava M. S-adenosyl methionine (SAMe) augmentation of serotonin reuptake inhibitors for antidepressant nonresponders with major depressive disorder. American Journal of Psychiatry. 2010;167(8):942-948.

Mischoulon D, Fava M. Role of S-adenosyl-L-methionine in the treatment of depression: a review of the evidence. American Journal of Clinical Nutrition. 2002;76(5):1158S-1161S.

On the HOPE-2 trial and CSPPT — homocysteine reduction and stroke prevention:

Lonn E, Yusuf S, Arnold MJ, et al. Homocysteine lowering with folic acid and B vitamins in vascular disease. New England Journal of Medicine. 2006;354(15):1567-1577.

Huo Y, Li J, Qin X, et al. Efficacy of folic acid therapy in primary prevention of stroke among adults with hypertension in China: the CSPPT randomized clinical trial. JAMA. 2015;313(13):1325-1335.

On the Horvath epigenetic clock and methylation aging:

Horvath S. DNA methylation age of human tissues and cell types. Genome Biology. 2013;14(10):R115.

Fiorito G, Polidoro S, Dugué PA, et al. Social adversity and epigenetic aging: a multi-cohort study on socioeconomic differences in peripheral blood DNA methylation. Scientific Reports. 2017;7(1):16266.

Cluster 10: The Detoxification Network

On CYP450 genetic variants and pharmacogenomics:

Ingelman-Sundberg M. Genetic polymorphisms of cytochrome P450 2D6 (CYP2D6): clinical consequences, evolutionary aspects and functional diversity. Pharmacogenomics Journal. 2005;5(1):6-13.

Zanger UM, Schwab M. Cytochrome P450 enzymes in drug metabolism: regulation of gene expression, enzyme activities, and impact of genetic variation. Pharmacology & Therapeutics. 2013;138(1):103-141.

On beta-glucuronidase and estrogen recycling:

Kwa M, Plottel CS, Blaser MJ, Adams S. The intestinal microbiome and estrogen receptor-positive female breast cancer. Journal of the National Cancer Institute. 2016;108(8):djw029.

On GSTM1 and GSTT1 null genotypes and cancer risk:

Ye Z, Song H. Glutathione S-transferase polymorphisms (GSTM1, GSTP1 and GSTT1) and the risk of acute leukemia: a systematic review and meta-analysis. European Journal of Cancer. 2005;41(7):980-989.

On phase I/phase II imbalance and reactive intermediates:

Guengerich FP. Cytochrome P450s and other enzymes in drug metabolism and toxicity. AAPS Journal. 2006;8(1):E101-E111.

Cluster 11: The Amino Acid Foundation

On mTOR, leucine threshold, and age-related blunting of muscle protein synthesis:

Wall BT, Hamer HM, de Vries A, et al. Leucine co-ingestion improves post-prandial muscle protein accretion in elderly men. Clinical Nutrition. 2013;32(3):412-419.

Devries MC, Phillips SM. Supplemental protein in support of muscle mass and health: advantage whey. Journal of Food Science. 2015;80 Suppl 1:A8-A15.

On PDCAAS and DIAAS protein quality scoring:

FAO. Dietary Protein Quality Evaluation in Human Nutrition: Report of an FAO Expert Consultation. FAO Food and Nutrition Paper 92. FAO; 2013.

On glycine synthesis capacity and deficit:

Meléndez-Hevia E, De Paz-Lugo P, Cornish-Bowden A, Cárdenas ML. A weak link in metabolism: the metabolic capacity for glycine biosynthesis does not satisfy the need for collagen synthesis. Journal of Biosciences. 2009;34(6):853-872.

On taurine, cardiovascular function, and depletion in vegans:

Yamori Y, Liu L, Ikeda K, et al. Distribution of twenty-four hour urinary taurine excretion and association with ischemic heart disease mortality in 24 populations of 16 countries: results from the WHO-CARDIAC study. Hypertension Research. 2001;24(4):453-457.

Wójcik OP, Koenig KL, Zeleniuch-Jacquotte A, et al. The potential protective effects of taurine on coronary heart disease.

Atherosclerosis. 2010;208(1):19-25.

On glutamine in surgical and critical care:

Wischmeyer PE, Dhaliwal R, McCall M, Ziegler TR, Heyland DK. Parenteral glutamine supplementation in critical illness: a systematic review. Critical Care. 2014;18(2):R76.

Cluster 12: The Fat-Soluble Foundations

On BCMO1 genetic variants and beta-carotene conversion efficiency:

Lietz G, Oxley A, Leung W, Hesketh J. Single nucleotide polymorphisms upstream from the β-carotene 15,15'-monoxygenase gene influence provitamin A conversion efficiency in female volunteers. Journal of Nutrition. 2012;142(1):161S-165S. On retinol teratogenicity and upper intake limits in pregnancy: Rothman KJ, Moore LL, Singer MR, et al. Teratogenicity of high vitamin A intake. New England Journal of Medicine. 1995;333(21):1369-1373.

On vitamin D as a steroid hormone and the VDR — 2000+ gene targets:

Holick MF. Vitamin D deficiency. New England Journal of Medicine. 2007;357(3):266-281.

Deeb KK, Trump DL, Johnson CS. Vitamin D signaling pathways in cancer: potential for anticancer therapeutics. Nature Reviews Cancer. 2007;7(9):684-700.

On vitamin D deficiency prevalence globally:

Cashman KD, Dowling KG, Škrabáková Z, et al. Vitamin D deficiency in Europe: pandemic? American Journal of Clinical Nutrition. 2016;103(4):1033-1044.

On vitamin K2 (MK-7) pharmacokinetics and the Rotterdam Study:

Geleijnse JM, Vermeer C, Grobbee DE, et al. Dietary intake of menaquinone is associated with a reduced risk of coronary heart disease: the Rotterdam Study. Journal of Nutrition. 2004;134(11):3100-3105.

Schurgers LJ, Vermeer C. Differential lipoprotein transport pathways of K-vitamins in healthy subjects. Biochimica et Biophysica Acta. 2002;1570(1):27-32.

On tocotrienols and their distinct biological properties:

Sen CK, Khanna S, Roy S. Tocotrienols: vitamin E beyond tocopherols. Life Sciences. 2006;78(18):2088-2098.

On RXR as nuclear receptor hub — vitamin A and D interaction:

Mark M, Ghyselinck NB, Chambon P. Function of retinoid nuclear receptors. Annual Review of Pharmacology and Toxicology. 2006;46:451-480.

Cluster 13: The Essential Fatty Acids

On the omega-3 index as a biomarker of cardiovascular risk:

Harris WS, von Schacky C. The Omega-3 Index: a new risk factor for death from coronary heart disease? Preventive Medicine. 2004;39(1):212-220.

Harris WS, Del Gobbo L, Tintle NL. The Omega-3 Index and relative risk for coronary heart disease mortality: estimation from 10 cohort studies. Atherosclerosis. 2017;262:51-54.

On DHA and neuronal membrane function in development and aging:

Innis SM. Dietary omega 3 fatty acids and the developing brain. Brain Research. 2008;1237:35-43.

Kidd PM. Omega-3 DHA and EPA for cognition, behavior, and mood: clinical findings and structural-functional synergies with cell membrane phospholipids. Alternative Medicine Review. 2007;12(3):207-227.

On the historical shift in omega-3:omega-6 ratio in Western diets:

Simopoulos AP. The importance of the ratio of omega-6/omega-3 essential fatty acids. Biomedicine & Pharmacotherapy. 2002;56(8):365-379.

Blasbalg TL, Hibbeln JR, Ramsden CE, Majchrzak SF, Rawlings RR. Changes in consumption of omega-3 and omega-6 fatty acids in the United States during the 20th century. American Journal of Clinical Nutrition. 2011;93(5):950-962.

On 4-hydroxynonenal (4-HNE) from heated seed oils:

Csala M, Kardon T, Legeza B, et al. On the role of 4-hydroxynonenal in health and disease. Biochimica et Biophysica Acta. 2015;1852(5):826-838.

Grootveld M, Percival BC, Leenders J, Edgar M. Potential adverse public health effects afforded by the ingestion of dietary lipid oxidation product toxins: significance of fried food sources. Nutrients. 2020;12(4):974.

On the REDUCE-IT trial — high-dose EPA and cardiovascular events:

Bhatt DL, Steg PG, Miller M, et al. Cardiovascular risk reduction with icosapentaenoic acid for hypertriglyceridemia. New England Journal of Medicine. 2019;380(1):11-22.

On trans fatty acids and cardiovascular disease:

Mozaffarian D, Katan MB, Ascherio A, Stampfer MJ, Willett WC. Trans fatty acids and cardiovascular disease. New England Journal of Medicine. 2006;354(15):1601–1613.

Cluster 14: The Supporting Cast — Protective Compounds

On Nrf2, Keap1, and ARE-driven cytoprotective gene expression:

Itoh K, Wakabayashi N, Katoh Y, et al. Keap1 represses nuclear activation of antioxidant responsive elements by Nrf2 through binding to the amino-terminal Neh2 domain. Genes & Development. 1999;13(1):76-86.

Dinkova-Kostova AT, Holtzclaw WD, Kensler TW. The role of Keap1 in cellular protective responses. Chemical Research in Toxicology. 2005;18(12):1779-1791.

On sulforaphane as the most potent dietary Nrf2 activator and phase II enzyme induction:

Zhang Y, Talalay P, Cho CG, Posner GH. A major inducer of anticarcinogenic protective enzymes from broccoli: isolation and elucidation of structure. Proceedings of the National Academy of Sciences. 1992;89(6):2399-2403.

Egner PA, Chen JG, Zarth AT, et al. Rapid and sustainable detoxication of airborne pollutants by broccoli sprout beverage: results of a randomized clinical trial in China. Cancer Prevention Research. 2014;7(8):813-823.

On quercetin as a zinc ionophore and intracellular zinc transport:

Dabbagh-Bazarbachi H, Clergeaud G, Quesada IM, Ortiz M, O'Sullivan CK, Fernández-Larrea JB. Zinc ionophore activity of quercetin and epigallocatechin-gallate: from Hepa 1-6 cells to a liposome model. Journal of Agricultural and Food Chemistry. 2014;62(32):8085-8093.

On lutein and zeaxanthin in macular pigment and the AREDS2 trial:

AREDS2 Research Group. Lutein + zeaxanthin and omega-3 fatty acids for age-related macular degeneration: the Age-Related Eye Disease Study 2 (AREDS2) randomized clinical trial. JAMA. 2013;309(19):2005-2015.

Bernstein PS, Li B, Vachali PP, et al. Lutein, zeaxanthin, and meso-zeaxanthin: the basic and clinical science underlying carotenoid-based nutritional interventions against ocular disease. Progress in Retinal and Eye Research. 2016;50:34-66.

On lycopene bioavailability, cis-isomer conversion by cooking, and prostate accumulation:

Gann PH, Ma J, Giovannucci E, et al. Lower prostate cancer risk in men with elevated plasma lycopene levels: results of a prospective analysis. Cancer Research. 1999;59(6):1225-1230.

Stahl W, Sies H. Lycopene: a biologically important carotenoid for humans? Archives of Biochemistry and Biophysics. 1996;336(1):1-9.

On bromelain and systemic anti-inflammatory and fibrinolytic effects:

Maurer HR. Bromelain: biochemistry, pharmacology and medical use. Cellular and Molecular Life Sciences. 2001;58(9):1234-1245.

On nattokinase fibrinolytic activity and cardiovascular effects:

Sumi H, Hamada H, Tsushima H, Mihara H, Muraki H. A novel fibrinolytic enzyme (nattokinase) in the vegetable cheese Natto; a typical and popular soybean food in the Japanese diet. Experientia. 1987;43(10):1110-1111.

Kim JY, Gum SN, Paik JK, et al. Effects of nattokinase on blood pressure: a randomized, controlled trial. Hypertension

Research. 2008;31(8):1583-1588.

On spermidine, autophagy induction via EP300 inhibition, and the prospective mortality data:

Eisenberg T, Knauer H, Schauer A, et al. Induction of autophagy by spermidine promotes longevity. Nature Cell Biology. 2009;11(11):1305-1314.

Kiechl S, Pechlaner R, Willeit P, et al. Higher spermidine intake is linked to lower mortality: a prospective population-based study. American Journal of Clinical Nutrition. 2018;108(2):371-380.

On inositol in PCOS, insulin signaling, and obsessive-compulsive spectrum conditions:

Unfer V, Carlomagno G, Dante G, Facchinetti F. Effects of myo-inositol in women with PCOS: a systematic review of randomized controlled trials. Gynecological Endocrinology. 2012;28(7):509-515.

Fux M, Levine J, Aviv A, Belmaker RH. Inositol treatment of obsessive-compulsive disorder. American Journal of Psychiatry. 1996;153(9):1219-1221.

On MSM, organic sulfur, and randomized trial evidence in osteoarthritis:

Kim LS, Axelrod LJ, Howard P, Buratovich N, Waters RF. Efficacy of methylsulfonylmethane (MSM) in osteoarthritis pain of the knee: a pilot clinical trial. Osteoarthritis and Cartilage. 2006;14(3):286-294.

On I3C, DIM, estrogen metabolism, and the 2:16 hydroxyoestrone ratio:

Bradlow HL, Telang NT, Sepkovic DW, Osborne MP. 2-hydroxyestrone: the 'good' estrogen. Journal of

Endocrinology. 1996;150 Suppl:S259-265.

Michnovicz JJ, Adlercreutz H, Bradlow HL. Changes in levels of urinary estrogen metabolites after oral indole-3-carbinol treatment in humans. Journal of the National Cancer Institute. 1997;89(10):718-723.

On sunlight, UVB-derived nitric oxide, and blood pressure reduction independent of vitamin D:

Liu D, Fernandez BO, Hamilton A, et al. UVA irradiation of human skin vasodilates arterial vasculature and lowers blood pressure independently of nitric oxide synthase. Journal of Investigative Dermatology. 2014;134(7):1839-1846.

On near-infrared photobiomodulation, cytochrome c oxidase, and mitochondrial ATP production:

Hamblin MR. Mechanisms and mitochondrial redox signaling in photobiomodulation. Photochemistry and Photobiology. 2018;94(2):199-212.

Karu TI. Mitochondrial signaling in mammalian cells activated by red and near-IR radiation. Photochemistry and Photobiology. 2008;84(5):1091-1099.

On circadian entrainment by morning light, melanopsin, the suprachiasmatic nucleus, and metabolic consequences of circadian disruption:

Provencio I, Rodriguez IR, Jiang G, Hayes WP, Moreira EF, Rollag MD. A novel human opsin in the inner retina. Journal of Neuroscience. 2000;20(2):600-605.

Roenneberg T, Merrow M. The circadian clock and human health. Current Biology. 2016;26(10):R432-443.

Berson DM, Dunn FA, Takao M. Phototransduction by retinal ganglion cells that set the circadian clock. Science. 2002;295(5557):1070-1073.

About the Author

Ravi Chimakurthy grew up in Eluru, a small town on the southeastern coast of India, and has lived and worked across Australia and the United States. An engineer by training and systems analyst by profession, he has spent two decades in the literature doing what the demands of modern clinical practice rarely permit: asking why so many people remain persistently unwell and dependent on multiple medications. That question became this book.

He brings to nutrition the instincts of a systems thinker — mapping nutritional root causes rather than downstream symptoms of disease, questioning non-essential classifications and the industry bias that elevates a few nutrients while the rest go unexamined. His research draws from the primary literature and his own health journey — two decades of pattern recognition that led him to hypothesize the Invisible Famine Hypothesis.

He has watched how people — including himself — navigate a modern medical system better equipped to diagnose and manage disease than to prevent or resolve it. This book is his answer to that gap.

Sick, Spent, & 60 Nutrients Short is his debut work of science non-fiction. With this book, he hopes readers will start asking their clinicians Why — and be unwilling to settle for What.

He lives in Atlanta, Georgia, with his wife and two daughters.

www.ingramcontent.com/pod-product-compliance
Lightning Source LLC
LaVergne TN
LVHW100248210926
848480LV00003B/864